How to Take C

BACK

Also by the same Author
in UBSPD

all you need to know about

PAIN IN YOUR NECK

and how to get rid of it

How to Take Care of Your

BACK

Dr. P. S. Ramani

M.S. (Bom.); C.R.C.S. Neuro (LOND); M.Sc. Neuro (Eng); F.A.C.S. (USA); F.I.C.S. (USA)

UBSPD
UBS Publishers' Distributors Ltd.
New Delhi Mumbai Bangalore Madras
Calcutta Patna Kanpur London

UBS Publishers' Distributors Ltd.
5 Ansari Road, New Delhi-110 002
Mumbai Bangalore Madras
Calcutta Patna Kanpur London

Copyright © 1994 Dr. P. S. Ramani

1996 Edition

Dr. P. S. Ramani asserts the moral right to be identified
as the author of this work.

All rights reserved. No part of this publication may be reproduced or transmitted in any form or by any means, electronic or mechanical including photocopying, recording, or any information storage and retrieval system, without permission in writing from the publisher.

Cover Design : UBS Art Studio

Printed at Rajkamal Electric Press, Delhi

YOUR MANUAL ON

* PREVENTION OF INJURY TO BACK

* CHOICE OF EXERCISE PROGRAMME

* MANAGEMENT OF BACKACHE

* KEEPING BACK IN SHAPE

CONTENTS

		Page
1.	Preliminary	1
2.	Introduction	3
3.	**Part-I** The Structure and Functions of Spine	7
4.	**Part-II** Mechanism, Prediction and Prevention of Backpain	13
5.	**Part-III** Exercises, Fitness, Do's and Dont's Keep Your Back in Shape	29
6.	**Part-IV** Essential Presenting Features of Backpain and Sciatica	39
7.	**Part-V** Guidelines for Management * Home Remedies * Consultations * Surgery * Fitness	45
8.	**Supplement:** Exercises To Keep the Back and the Body Healthy (To be carried out at home)	59

YOUR MANUAL ON YOUR BACK

THIS book is intended to give latest up-to-date information on how to keep one's back in good shape, what to do when there is back pain and in turn it tells you how to keep your back in shape and thus remain physically healthy.

Part I : Explains the structure and functions of spine in a very simple language and with only basic concepts. It gives basic knowledge about various curves and postures.

Part II : Explains how back can get injured and how to prevent it. It also explains the prepondering factors which lead to backache and gives useful tips on prevention of backsprains.

Part III : Concentrates on day to day practical tips so that the back can be kept in shape. It also gives a set of select exercises to be done to prevent back pain and to keep it in shape after back pain has resolved. The set of exercises is printed at the end as supplement.

Part IV : Explains essential symptoms and presenting features of backpain. It also explains the behaviour of a patient with backache and sciatica in the house.

Part V : Tells you what to do when one is afflicted with back pain. At first practical tips on home remedies are given. Then the indications to consult a doctor are outlined. When surgery is required the manual tells you how to keep your morale high. It also gives useful practical suggestions.

Consider this as your manual for good health. It will ultimately motivate you to keep your back in proper shape and feel proud about it.

INTRODUCTION

BACKACHE is as prevalent in our society as headache or common cold. It is also a fact that backache is more often ignored. Many people tolerate backache with the belief that modern medicine has little to offer. It can be transient or a reflection of underlying disease which if neglected can ultimately disable an individual and force him into early retirement.

IT CAN AFFECT YOU:

It afflicts all groups of people from workers in industry to executives in the big business houses, from housewives at home to elderly in the ashrams. Taken together backache accounts for more man-hours lost, more man-hours spent in the hospital and many man-hours of lost pleasure at home and outside than any other condition. Backache is also known as backpain or back sprain. Lumbago is usually a sprain in the lower part of the back or lumbar spine. Although usually associated with activity such as lifting a heavy box, it can also occur during rest or relaxation. In fact more severe backaches have originated during sleep as a result of lying in a wrong posture.

TREATMENT IS EFFECTIVE:

In recent times the treatment of backache has improved significantly. Most patients thus afflicted can improve with bed rest and home medicines. For the small minority who need it, the surgery on the spine today has become very safe and effective when performed by experts. In fact in a given case of herniated or prolapsed lumbar intervertebral disc, the surgery with microlumbar discectomy has become not only effective but so swift that patient can be discharged from the hospital within 24 hours making it a "Come today Go tomorrow" surgery.

PATTERN OF BACKPAIN:

As always, prevention of backache is preferable to cure. Valuable and useful advice is offered in this book on how to keep the back strong and healthy and resist routine attacks of back sprain.

IT HAPPENED TO ME:

I had gone on a holiday to Lonavala. While coming back I was driving a Maruti car. The traffic was heavy. It took a long time to reach home. My back had become stiff. I got out of the car on reaching home and was walking up to the lift when my nephew called me to show his new tricycle. I went up to him and lifted this four year old hefty boy bending awkwardly over his tricycle. It did not occur to me that I should bend my knees. I thought I was strong. After playing with the boy for a couple of minutes, I started walking upto the lift. The shoe lace was loose and I bent to tie it. I could not get up. I felt as if someone had poked me in the back with an iron rod (hot). Somehow I straightened myself and managed to reach my flat. The next day was worse. I took rest and took analgesics, anti-inflammatory drugs, muscle relaxants and hot fomentation.

After two days I tried to get out of bed with the help of a corset. One full week passed before I started feeling better. I cursed myself for not following simple instructions that I everyday, as a spinal surgeon, taught to my patients. In a way I was happy that I could realise what my patients were suffering from.

It is a cruel irony that as a spinal surgeon I have to stand and bend forwards for hours together to do spinal surgery. Something a patient of backache should not do. I sometimes feel that while trying to relieve patients' backache I ruin my own back by standing and bending forward for several hours during surgery. Something I always teach my patients not to do. Since this episode I now practice what I preach.

At the end of each surgery I do religiously a set of exercises to keep my back strong and mobile, free from stiffness that usually creeps in after long hours of standing and bending forwards over surgery. I no longer bend forward to tie my lace without bending my knees and I no longer bend awkwardly over the tricycle to lift my nephew.

IT CAN HAPPEN TO YOU:

Mr. C. Tiwari was in his thirties. As a salesman he has been quite active running from one place to another and he always thought he was strong. He did not bother to follow simple principles of avoiding getting a backache. He was to get married. There were not many people in the family to help him with the marriage arrangements with the result that he had to do a lot of running about. So much so that by the morning of the day of wedding he was stiff in the back. Without showing any pang he went through the ritual of wedding. He bent forwards to say Namaskar to his father in law. He felt the same pang in the back that I had felt in my back. He could not get up. He had to be bodily lifted up and taken to the nursing home instead of going to his honeymoon. Mr. Tiwari was very depressed. The thought that was haunting him all the time "Will doctor say that I will need surgery?" By and large the chances are that Mr. Tiwari will not require surgery provided he follows simple instructions about care of the back and does not abuse it unnecessarily.

DO NOT ABUSE YOUR BACK:

Mr. C.Y. Rajesh is an executive in a reputed firm in the city of Bombay. He is 44 years old and holds a responsible position in the company. He has to work late hours in the night.

Ten years back he suffered from backache. He had consulted me then and examination and investigations had shown that he in fact has suffered from prolapsed lumbar intervertebral disc that was not too big to require surgery. I had warned him then that if he followed simple instructions about back care perhaps he may never need an operation in spite of the fact that he suffered from prolapsed lumbar intervertebral disc causing backache. Mr. Rajesh takes good care of his back. Ten years have passed. He has not required surgery. He wears soft sole shoes instead of high heel stiff leather shoes and in the evening when work is over he sends his car away with the chauffeur and walks home from Nariman Point to Malabar Hill.

RESPECT YOUR BACK:

Mr. K.C. Dalal is a finance consultant. He was very fond of jogging and walking and hiking. He did suffer from a large prolapsed disc and I had to operate upon his back. He was dejected. He thought he will have to give up his jogging and hiking. I reassured him and put him through the back mobilisation and strengthening exercises. Mr. Dalal started feeling strength once again in his back and with it his morale started rising. Exactly on the first anniversary of surgery he wrote to me a letter saying "Dear Doctor, for the tenth time today I climbed Matheran after the operation at the age of 46 years". I am writing this letter rather than telephone to you so that you can show this letter to your innumerable patients about the wonders of keeping the back in shape even after surgery.

PART – I

THE STRUCTURE AND FUNCTIONS OF SPINE

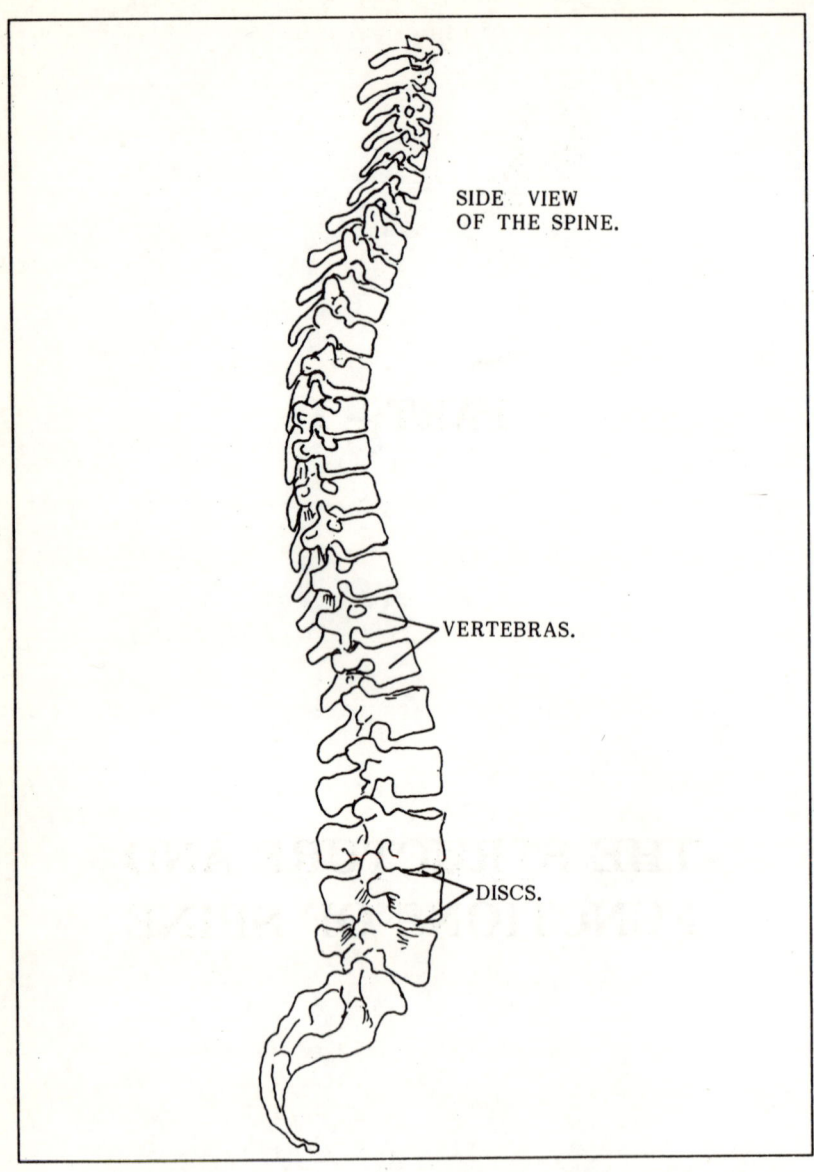

Fig. 1: The whole human spine. It is gently curved to provide maximum flexibility while providing all the strength. It has seven vertebrae in the cervical region 12 in the thoracic region and five in the lumbar region. The sacral 5 vertebrae are fused together to form the sacrum and at the end is the tail bone the coccyx.

BASIC KNOWLEDGE OF SPINE

The Structure of Spine:

THE human spine is also known as vertebral column because it appears straight and upright when viewed from the front or back. It is made of small pieces called vertebrae stacked neatly on one another like wooden blocks and then it is divided into portions such as cervical, dorsal, lumbar and sacral spinal regions. The solid portion of each vertebra in front is known as body. From the body two prong like pedicles on either side enclose a space and forms the canal through which passes the spinal cord. The two prongs meet at the back to form the spinous process. This knob can be felt under the skin at the back like a line of beads.

On either side of the spinous process are the facet joints which serve as hinges between the vertebra above and the one below. The function of these joints is to provide smooth gliding movements and restrict the range of motion (ROM) when it goes beyond limits. Each facet joint is covered by joint capsule which lubricates the joint through synovial fluid. Facet joint is not designed to carry excessive body weight. The two transverse processes on either side of the vertebra are like two wings of the plane and helps to balance the vertebra in position.

The Intervertebral Disc:

One disc is interposed between two vertebral bodies. It is like a dunlop cushion. It is made up of inner spongy portion called the nucleus pulposus and an outer firm ring of fibrous tissue called the annulus. Under abnormal stresses there is disruption of the outer annulus and the central nucleus pushes

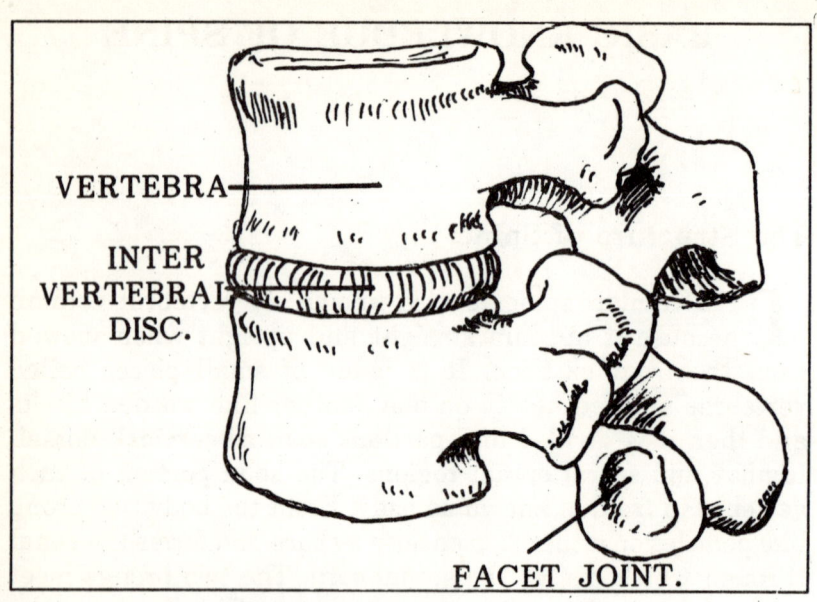

Fig. 2

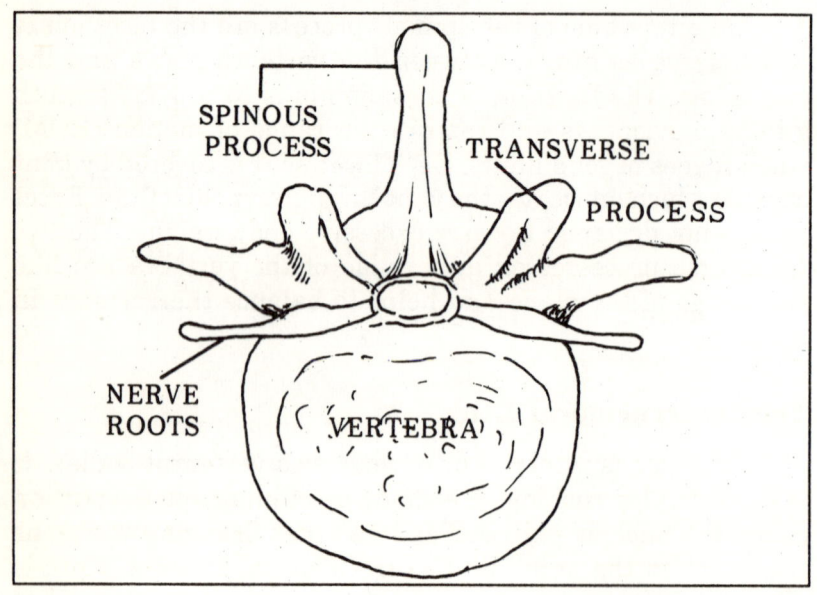

Fig. 3

itself out with great pressure through the rent in the annulus and thus lay the foundation for prolapsed lumbar intervertebral disc.

A given disc is subject to daily wear and tear so that with passing years the disc wears out and becomes dry.

Typically a disc can take lot of pressure, upto 1000 kg. It can tolerate a lot of abuse and resist injury. It is self lubricating. However, it cannot repair itself once it is torn, consequently although the pain of sprain can be relieved, the damage done to the disc cannot be repaired and has real consequence for life.

The blood supply to the disc stops at the age of 20 years. After that it depends on daily activity like spinal exercises, jogging, aerobic exercises, etc. to lubricate itself and stay healthy.

The perfect spine appears straight and upright from the back or from the front view. The side view reveals that it is actually not straight at all. It form as S shape with a slight curve in the low back and another near the neck. It is the forward lordotic curve in the neck that makes the neck tall and beautiful allowing ladies to wear nice jewellery round the neck and men to wear smart ties and broad collared shirts. It really does make one look smart. Besides, the curves allow the spine to carry great body weight and at the same time generate incredible lifting force.

The lumbar portion of the spine made up of five vertebrae is the seat of backache and sciatica as it has two important functions to perform. It has to be extremely mobile to be able to do the break dance and at the same time it has to transmit the heavy weight of the body to the legs. The last two vertebrae bear the greatest stress while transmitting the weight and thus prolapsed disc is most common at these two places.

The Muscles:

It is believed that most back spains result from injury to the back muscles. The spinal muscles lie vertically on either side of the mid-line at the back around the bony vertebrae. Like vertebrae each individual muscles is small and spans at the most two or three vertebrae. The abdominal muscles play an important role in maintaining posture and strength of the spine. If abdominal muscles become lax and one develops the so called prosperity paunch the spine arches forwards in sway back pain. The quardriceps muscles of the thigh are the powerhouse of the body. The stronger a person's legs the less is the load transmitted to the spine. By proper posturing, the burden of lifting should be transmitted to quadriceps in the legs thus sparing the spine. The spinal muscles are more prone to go into spasm, under stress. If the muscles will not work, the extra load will be transmitted to the ligaments which under sustained pressure become lax and loose their ability to maintain proper posture. As you see all the structures in the spine i.e. the vertebrae, the discs, joints, ligaments, muscles and nerves together make the healthy spine the workhorse of the body. Hence remember! if spine is healthy the body will definitely be healthy.

PART - II

MECHANISM PREDICTION AND PREVENTION OF BACK PAIN

CAUSES AND PREVENTION OF BACK PAIN

WHAT CAUSES THE BACKPAIN:

THE spine with its intricate series of bones, joints, ligament and muscles is in fact extremely resistant to injuries. But it needs to be looked after. The muscles need to be toned, the joints need to be kept well lubricated and smooth. All this can be achieved by organised motion. The spine needs motion to retain motion. The motion lubricates the joints and tones the muscles so that they are less prone to strain and result in wear and tear not related to age.

Unfortunately many back problems develop because most of the people do not service their spinal engine regularly. It is believed that four out of every five people in a given urban society will experience back pain at some time in their lives. Many back problems develop because our sedentary life styles allow our backs to get out of condition.

UNUSUAL ACTIVITY:

Spine must be regularly toned. A sudden spurt in activity for a unserviced spine can also lead to backpain and sicatica. Imagine an executive working through the whole week in his office lifting nothing more heavier than his smoking pipe or expensive fountain pen suddenly decides to drive himself to Pune on Saturday to attend the Derby Race on Sunday. He is bound to sprain his muscles and ligaments in the back and lay foundation for chronic backache.

OCCUPATIONAL BACKPAIN:

Backpain could be a serious problem among working people. It is most common between the ages of thirty and fifty

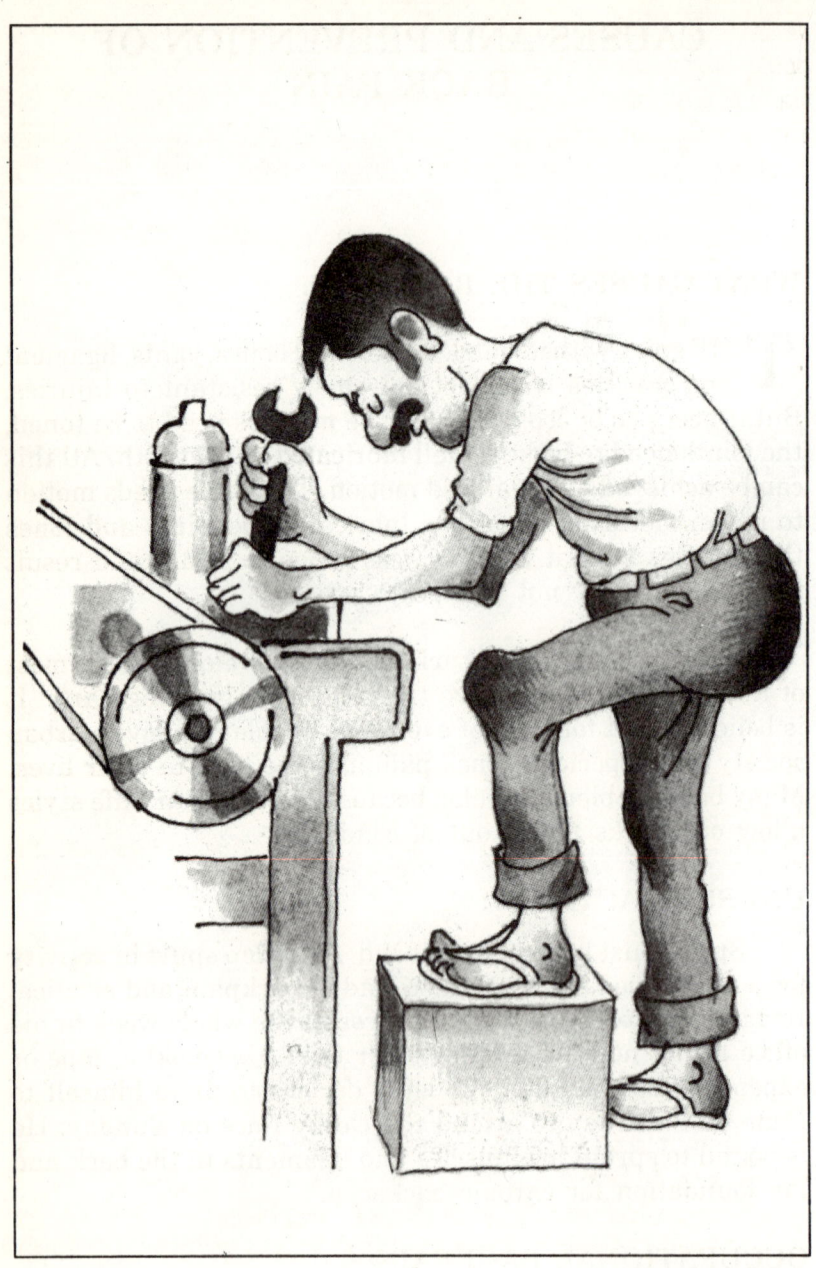

Fig. 4: While working a low stool under one foot helps to bend the knee and keep the spine straight. A more relaxed position.

years with both men and women being equally affected. Certain occupations have higher risk of back pain. Garbage collectors have the highest risk of having backache on the job when they repeatedly perform the most difficult motion of throwing a garbage basket into a moving truck. Many back problems occur not from falls from ladder or from scaffolding but from lifting inappropriately something which normally should have been within their capability. Nobody likes to have backache. But it comes like an unwelcome visitor at most inappropriate times without much warning. It remains for a long time and once the friendship is developed it returns very frequently.

SOURCES OF BACKPAIN:

Although the sources of backpain can be varied, eighty per cent of the times the cause can be pinpointed either to muscles, the intervertebral discs or the joints.

Muscle Sprain:

Normally the muscles of the back contract and relax in rhythm with the movements of the back. When the muscle is under abnormal strain it goes into spasm tensing up to a point that it becomes hard as lump. The muscle can cramp due to overwork or if there is a problem in the joint or even emotionally the muscle can cramp. Fortunately most of the times the sprain becomes better with home remedies such as fomentation analgesics and muscle relaxants.

Herniated (Prolapsed) Intervertebral Discs:

This is the second most common source of backpain and sciatica. As described above it is most common in the lowest two lumbar vertebrae. The herniated disc besides causing backache, also produces pressure on the nearby spinal nerves. Wear and tear with advancing years leads to degeneration in the annulus which then bulges more than normal in the spinal canal. Under stress the disc bulges significantly into the canal. It compresses the adjoining nerve and causes sciatic pain. A degenerated disc requires less force to bulge further.

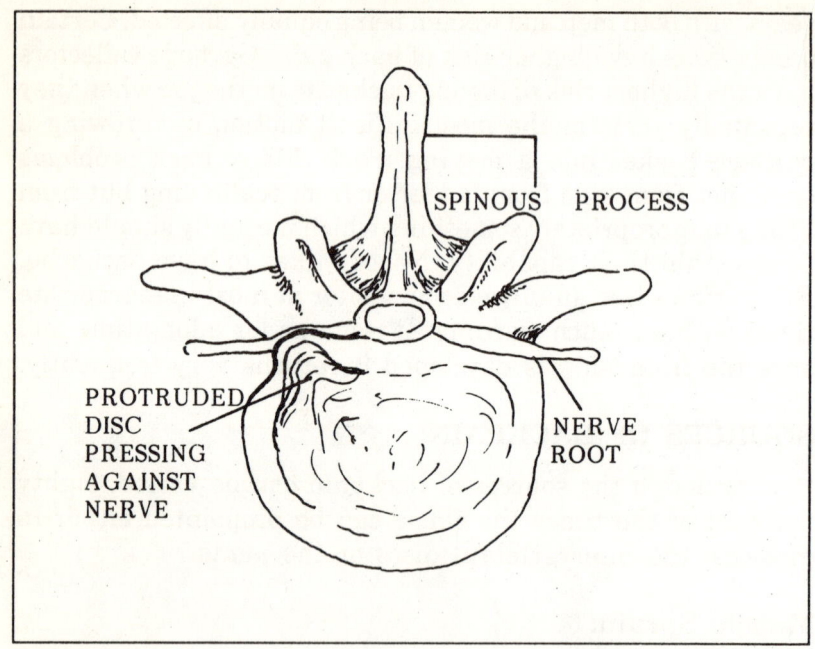

Fig. 5: Protruding intervertebral disc compressed the root as it comes out of the intervertebral forarmen giving rise to backache and sciatica.

Common example is the morning manouver. You are bending forwards near the sink and brushing the teeth. You cough forcefully to clear the throat or sneeze in this position and very often the degenerated disc herniates and causes pressure on the nerve forcing you to visit the doctor. Leg pain or sciatica is a common by-product of back pain.

Joints:

Facet joint must line precisely with those above and below. This helps the back to twist and bend with little friction of the bony surfaces. A sudden jerk or twist can sprain a facet joint and cause pain much like the pain in the knee joint sprain. By continued long term stress the capsule becomes stiff and rough and it loses its power to lubricate the joint and leads to chronic pain. This, in fact, is the common cause of chronic backpain.

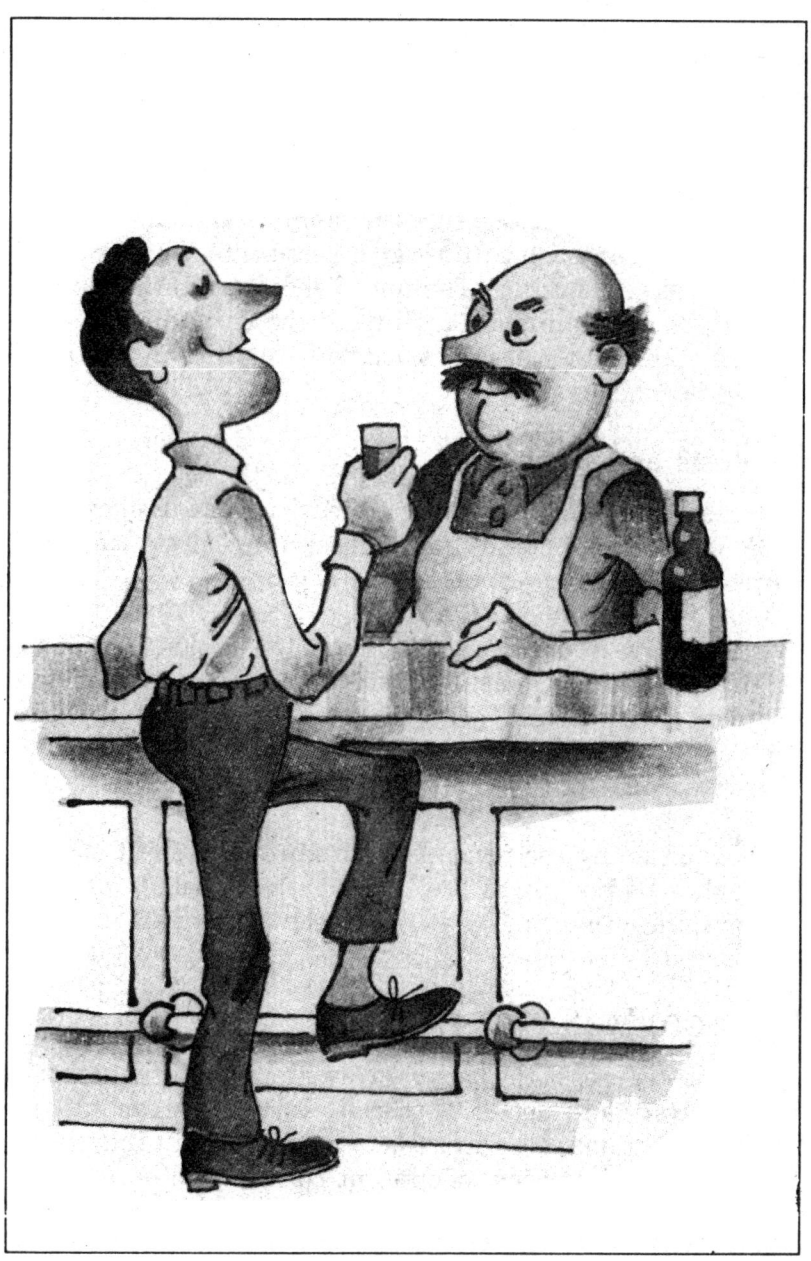
Fig. 6: Rails are provided in the bar to help one relax his spine while he is standing there for hours together drinking beer.

Given the whole spine, because of its vulnerability, most spinal problems occur in the lumbar region than anywhere else.

Other Causes of Backpain:

As viewed from the side the spine is S shaped. It has curvatures. These curvatures give posture to the body what is known as good posture. The spine needs constant disciplined activity to maintain good posture. If the curvatures become abnormal the person assumes bad posture which in turn gives rise to backache.

Lordosis and Kyphosis:

Lordosis refers to the forward curve of the lumbar spine when viewed from the side and kyphosis refers to the backward curve of the thoracic spine.

Excessive lordosis can be a congenital problem or problem related to certain elements of the spine. More often it is a postural problem and is more related to the presence of protruding abdomen. It produces stress on the joints and generate pain.

Maintaining the normal and natural curve of the spine through good posture is the best way to distribute the load on the spine evenly among all the structures that are designed to carry it.

LESS COMMON CAUSES:

Other causes of the backpain are spinal stenosis, scoliosis, spondilolysis and spondilolisthesis. Instability can also be caused by trauma, arthritis, osteoporosis, etc. But they do not fall within the purview of present communication.

Backpain by Occupational Poor Posture:

Both at home and at work one gets into positions whether standing sitting or bending, that can trigger backpain.

The pressure produced in the disc and the spine changes with the position. Least pressure in produced on the spine in lying down position, flat on the back. As soon as we stand up, the pressure on the spine increases three times. Sitting is even worse than standing. When we lift a box weighing 15 to 20 kg the pressure on the disc increases to more than five times. But if we lift the same box improperly by bending over at the waist instead of bending the knees, the pressure is increased to over ten times.

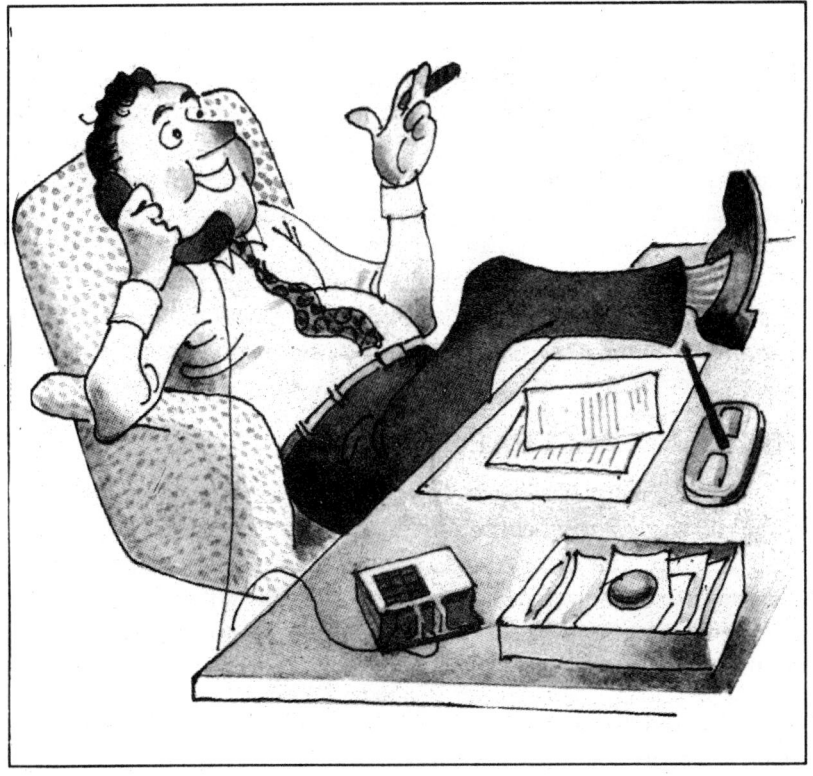

Fig. 7: Deconditioned muscles, overweight, protruding belly and bad posture is a prescription for backache and sciatica.

Poor posture also stretches the ligaments when a worker has to stay hunched to a work or factory assembly line for hours together. A weight lifted without warming up can certainly pull the ligaments and stretch the muscles and herniate an intervertebral disc.

Is Pain Different for Different People:

Yes. Indeed it is. Besides the complex nature of the spine different people have different thresholds for pain. The threshold of pain can be related to cultural factors, personality traits and even social and economic factors. In certain religious cults pain in fact can be an ecstasy.

A person with backache cannot go to work. It affects his psychological state of mind. He starts worrying about a million life problems like "Will I ever be all right to work again, Will I find a substitute job, Will the management agree for permanent light job, Will my wife still love me?" These questions invite depression to add to the backpain.

If a person had backpain over a long period of time, chances are he may, unknowingly, have become drugs dependant and now the doctor will have one more problem to resolve that of drug addiction.

MIND AND BACKPAIN:

And finally backpain is so intriguing that at times it is difficult to define and measure. At times it makes the doctor pull his hair out in trying to evolve a conscentious in a given patient with backpain. It could be extremely frustrating. Not surprisingly some doctors even refuse to see patients with chronic backpain.

Any doctor intensely desires to help the patient who is suffering. It becomes frustrating when he is not in a position to achieve it. He is just not able to relieve the backpain.

SPECIALISED CLINICS:

At some places in the city, today, where there are specialised clinics for backpain, while the spinal surgeon is concerned about the backpain the clinic itself focuses on the

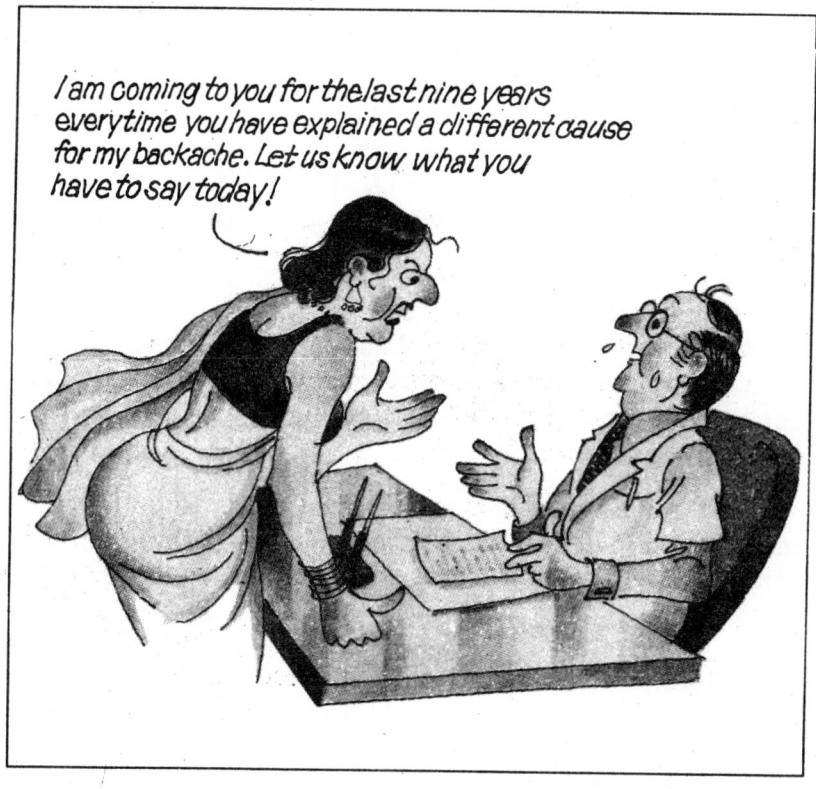

Fig. 8: Many times backache is nothing but tention from the mind which has slipped into the back.

functions that are affected by backpain. When a person does not look forward to go to work in the morning because of backpain and rather prefers to lie on the couch and watch television, the expectation of backpain can become a self fulfilling prophecy. The more he relaxes the more he looses initiative to go to work. The more he remains idle his capsules of the joints shrink, muscles become weak and aggravates the backpain. Over a period of time this type of downward trend can suck a person right down the drain.

SPORTS MEDICINE PRINCIPLE IN BACKPAIN:

Following backpain, many doctors rely heavily on bed rest and no activity to the muscles. Whereas in this book stress is laid, as in may places in the world, on activity after injury. The philosophy of encouraging activity after only two days of bed rest following backpain is stressed here.

This principle is obtained from sports medicine which has become so vibrant and active these days. Athletes today begin active rehabilitation and movements as early as possible after injury.

It may be stressed here that vast majority of backpain is caused by simple sprains and will cure itself if given enough time and proper exercise. Seventy per cent of the sprains will get better within three weeks and eighty per cent will get better by six weeks.

If the pain still persists then he needs to be specially investigated to determine more specific and perhaps surgical causes of the backpain like a prolapsed large intervertebral disc.

Can Backpain be Predicted? A New Concept:

This is in fact a new concept in the understanding of backpain and susceptibility of certain persons to get backpain. Ten years ago not many people knew what is cholesterol. Thanks to the active work done by cardiologists the world-over, today, all learned people understand what is cholesterol and its ill effects on the heart. People now routinely check for levels of cholesterol in the blood and if they are high, they immediately seek the cardiologist's advice to lower the cholesterol before it can produce deleterious effects on the heart.

On the same basis it is now possible in the field of spine care to determine a person's individual risk of back injury. Admittedly such tests are not easily available in this country.

COMPUTERISED ISOKINETIC TESTING (CIT):

The procedure is called Computerised Isokinetic Testing. Through this investigation the spine specialist can measure the strength of a person's back and get a pretty good picture of whether the person has back injury waiting to happen.

The Procedure:

In sitting position the person extends backwards and then forwards. This is done without using any resistance. The resistance is produced in direct proportion to the amount of torque created by the person. The stronger the back, more is the resistance and more is the torque registered on the computer. The computer than reads his abdominal and back muscle strength and compares it with the average figures readily available in the computer matching it with the body weight. It is measured in foot-pounds. The ratio between the extensor back muscles and abdominal muscles should be at least 3:2. The extensors of the spine should be able to produce a torque equivalent to this body weight.

How Do People Measure on This Test:

It is now realised that mine workers, fisherfolk, long distance runners and atheletes can produce torque of up to 200 per cent of their body weight. Peons, stenos, office clerks and office superintendents can hardly reach up to 70 per cent of their body weight and executives who indulge in recreational activities such as golf, swimming, playing tennis, etc. can reach very near the target.

Does it Help to Know Your Risk of Back Injury?

Yes. It does help to know the risk of back injury. Suppose the computerised isokinetic testing comes to about 75 per cent of the normal then one can start doing regular exercises to strengthen the extensors of the spine and at the same time observe the following precautions.

1. Do a warm up before lifting weights.
2. Do not get fatigued at the end of the day.
3. Do not try to lift something heavier than normal or do not lift weights that you are not normally accustomed to.

Desk Job and Backache:

Sitting for hours together doing desk job actually stresses

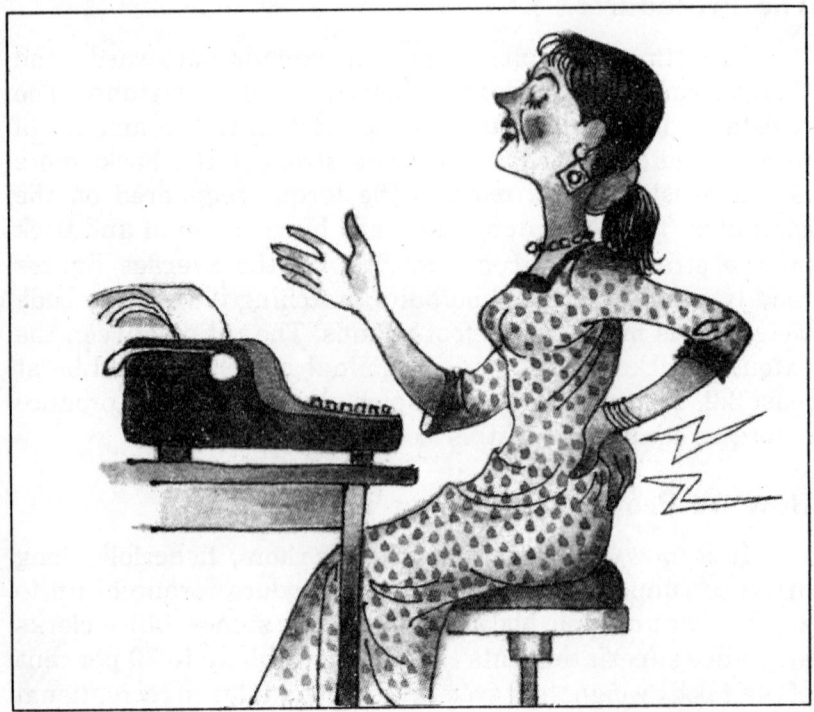

Fig. 9: Continuous day's work in one position without intermittently relaxing the back makes it sore and lays foundation for backache.

the back. It also does not help in any way to strengthen the back muscles. Intermittent walking, lifting small objects and bending throughout the day can become useful as an exercise maintenance programme.

Overweight:

It is now believed that having a protruding belly helps to pull the spine forwards out of alignment setting the stage for backpain. On the other hand strong abdominal muscles can definitely prevent back from many day-to-day assaults causing back pain.

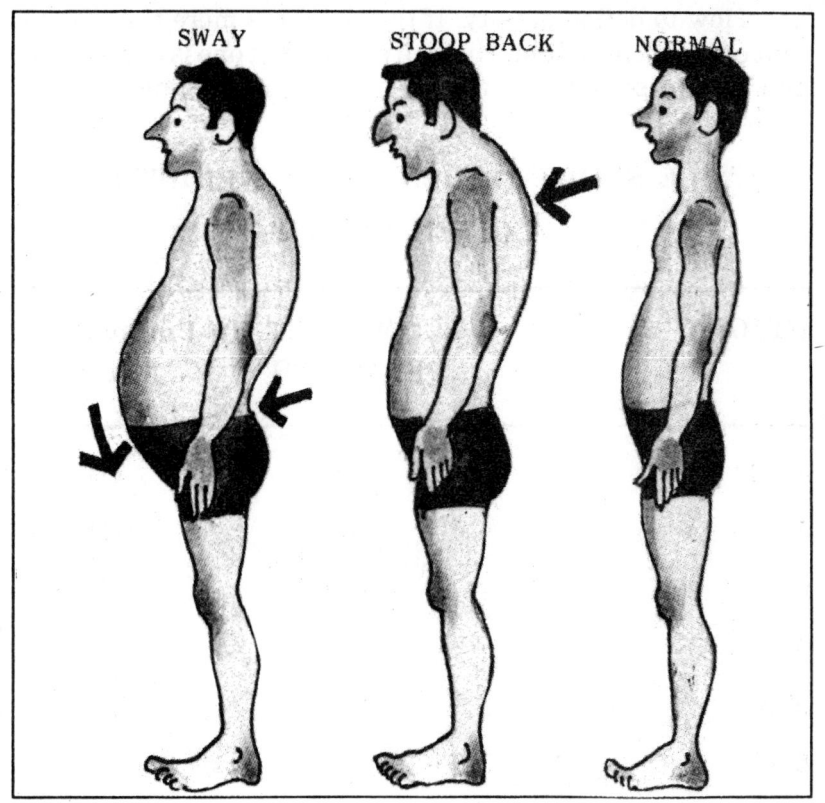

Fig. 10

Extra weight creates extra stress on the body and makes it difficult to maintain fitness programme.

How to define obesity: If the weight is more than 20 per cent of the ideal weight, clinically speaking, one is over-weight and should seek out a weight control programme.

TABLE SHOWING IDEAL BODY WEIGHT FOR A GIVEN HEIGHT

HEIGHT	WEIGHT (In Pounds) FEMALES	MALES
4' 11"	106	116
5' 0"	109	119
5' 1"	112	122
5' 2"	116	125
5' 3"	120	128
5' 4"	124	131
5' 5"	128	136
5' 6"	133	142
5' 7"	136	147
5' 8"	140	152
5' 9"	144	158
5' 10"	148	166
5' 11"	152	172
6' 0"	156	178

PART - III

* EXERCISES,
* FITNESS,
* DO'S AND DONT'S

KEEP YOUR BACK IN SHAPE

EXERCISE PROGRAMME FOR BACK CARE

SPORTS MEDICINE APPROACH:

AS described above the sports medicine approach should be used while recovering from back pain. The exercises should be continued even when the back pain has completely disappeared and if possible the set of exercises for keeping the back healthy should be started much before the back pain has started. It does not matter if one has done computerised testing or not, back-strengthening exercises can be started any day.

Sports medicine principles have shown that the former passive treatment of rest and inactivity makes recovery more difficult. Rapid wasting in the muscles makes it difficult and painful to return to activity early.

From physiological stand point of view the overall physical capacity of the cardiovascular and musculo skeletal system decreases rapidly with disuse. Even day-to-day activities seem difficult. The person then becomes more susceptible to strains and sprains. By forcing the person to return to activity the muscles and cardio-

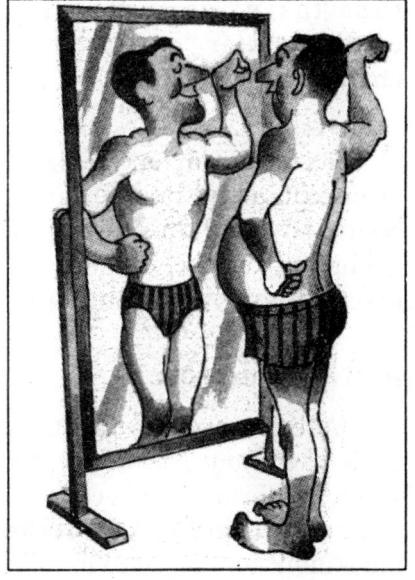

Fig. 11: A steady exercise programme can help one to get in shape and loose weight. It helps one to look better and get more work done.

vascular system have less time to atrophy and achieving full strength becomes easier and quicker.

NATURAL PAIN KILLERS:

The second benefit of exercises is that it stimulates body's natural pain killers, the endorphins and encephalins.

Endorphins are now known to be responsible for self-induced euphoria seen in runners. Endorphins raise the threshold for pain, enhances mood and fights depression. Without exercise, endorphins and other natural mood enhancers drop dramatically. Hence it is important to incorporate exercise into the daily routine to enjoy not only the benefits of strength and endurance but also to obtain the pain killing effect and mood elevating sensation.

Sports medicine approach is, in fact, a broad approach that takes into account physiological, psychological, cardiovascular, nutritional, biochemical, pathological and environmental factors.

Exercise is a very general term and it includes a variety of specific activities. To start with exercises must be done cautiously and carefully gradually increasing the activity depending on the endurance of the person. Exercises are essentially divided into four types.

Active Exercises:

Active exercises are those which are performed by the patient without assistance. The movements are less stressful when performed correctly. Active exercises require the co-ordination of muscles, joints and the nerves. Pain limits active movement and an individual's range of movement (ROM) can be assessed by the therapist. An individual can control his activity depending on pain and hence further injury can be avoided.

Resistive Exercises:

This exercises help the therapist assess the resistive power of the muscles, tendons, etc. More strength is required for resistive exercises which are usually done by the therapist but this added resistance helps to stress the muscles better than in active exercises.

The best example of resistive exercise is lifting a weight. More the strength in the muscles, the more is the weight that can be lifted. The increased delivery of blood in the resistive exercises allows tissues to stretch more and function more effectively with less pain and other related symptoms. With resistive exercises the cardiovascular system helps to flush out lactic acid that tend to accumulate in the muscles. Lactic acid is produced in the muscles in response to strain. It causes the muscle to fatigue when it is locally accumulated.

Passive Exercises:

These exercises are very light. They are usually performed on the back, soon after surgery, by the therapist while the patient is still in the hospital. The muscles are not contracted but the therapist passively and lightly lifts up the limbs. They are more used to increase the flexibility of the muscles and create confidence in the patient that by increasing flexibility the surgical wound is not going to have any complications or sutures are not going to give way.

Functional Exercises:

These exercises, particularly in the western countries, are performed as a form of occupational rehabilitation after surgery on the back. If a miner has undergone surgery on his back for prolapsed lumber intervertebral disc, after a reasonable period of safety, the therapist puts him through a set of rehabilitation exercises by simulating miner's activity at work. For warehouse worker the activity includes lifting boxes of various shapes and sizes with varying weights. Such exercises are extremely important to increase the confidence of the worker to return to work early with a smiling face if only he has the conviction to go to work early.

The Heart Rate:

While doing the exercise emphasis is laid on the enhancement of efficiency of the heart and lungs as together they deliver the much needed energy and oxygen to the exercising muscles. The efficiency of cardio-pulmonary system can be achieved by jogging, running or brisk walking. Walking is the best aerobic exercise in the programme of ideal back. Irrespective of the fact whether one runs, jogs or walks, the emphasis is on the duration and endurance rather than speed. A good pair of shoes is absolutely necessary. The goal is to raise the heart rate to a plateau. For a young healthy man it could be 180 beats per minute and for a man of 45 years it could be 140 beats per minute. (Individuals taking heart medicines must consult their doctor before starting the exercise).

Do Not Overdo:

How to know that one is not overdoing. While walking, after five to ten minutes one should be able to say five or six words without taking a deep breath. If he cannot do this then the intensity of aerobic is great.

If one does not like walking or jogging out in the playground, then he can achieve the same goal by using a stationery bicycle. The criticism for stationery bicycle lies in the fact that the weight of the body is taken away by the bike. The exercise may seem easy. Besides if one is suffering from prolapsed disc, sitting on the bicycle may not be comfortable.

Cool Down:

After completing the cardio-pulmonary toning allow one self to cool down to prevent blood from pooling in the legs. This may cause light headedness, dizziness, etc. The cool down period is for a minimum of three minutes. The cool down is complete when the heart rate returns to below 100 beats per minute.

The exercises for the back are illustrated in the supplement at then end of this book.

BENEFICIAL EFFECTS OF CERTAIN ACTIVITIES:

Swimming:

It is an aerobic exercise useful for the body. The propelling motions strengthen the shoulders and the upper body. Freestyle is good for strengthening spinal muscles but breast stroke may hyperextend the back causing pain. Use of life vest can allow sufficient range of motion and added weightlessness. Swimming can act as hydrotherapy to ease back into activity. For a patient who is recovering from back surgery, walking in the pool is a good resistive exercise to the legs and the body. For a more balanced development of the body, swimming must be combined with other spinal muscle-strengthening exercises.

Bicycling:

Bicycling is a good conditioner. It improves muscular endurance in the legs. Helps more to build thighs and legs. Prolonged flexion on the bicycle should be avoided. Seat should not be too high and handles too low. The points to be considered in the bicycle are:

(1) Size of the frame,
(2) Height of the seat,
(3) Comfortable position of the seat,
(4) Height of the handle bar in comparison with the height of the seat, and
(5) Reach to the handle bar from the seat.

In view of these points, it is preferable to buy a bicycle rather than hire one.

Running and Jogging:

Through this exercise the heart and the lungs are most benefited. The back muscles to some extent. Good pair of shoes are necessary to prevent damage from jarring effect of continually hitting on the ground. Shorter frequent runs are preferable to marathon runs. Running is a good aerobic fitness exercise. If one starts running after rehabilitation from backpain two things must be observed:

(1) Lumbosacral belt should be worn untill he feels confident.

(2) Abdominal muscles must be simultaneously strengthened.

Running helps to enhance mood, through release of natural endorphins.

Body-building:

The word body-building gives wrong impression as if one is trying for 'Bombay Shree' title. I would prefer to use the word Body Shaping. Gymnasium has no more remained the domain of body-builders. Most people, both males and females now flock to gyms merely for keeping the body in shape and in good health. This concept and the word 'Body Shaping' matches well with our concept of keeping the body and spine in good health. In big cities like Bombay most gymnasiums are crowded with females who want to keep body in shape. The key to success is to use weight lifting more frequently. The rule of thumb here shall be to use lighter weights and lift it up several times (25 times) instead of lifting a heavier weight only five times. Age should be a strong consideration while increasing the intensity of the workout. The greatest degeneration in the spine and the intervertebral discs occur between the ages of 25 and 35. One should remember that exercise is being done to keep the body in good health.

The Twisting Activity: Golf and Tennis:

Golf is such a sport that one can enjoy it the entire life.

Its slow speed, calculated activities does not produce too much stress on the body. On the other hand, it will be difficult to play tennis life long. High degree of body rotation, spine extension, the forehand, the back hand and the volleys all require high degree of quick and rapid generation of power that it becomes difficult to sustain the same power with advancing age.

However, both these sports involve twisting of the body. Many backsprains, tennis elbow and shoulder stiffness stem from the high degree of body rotation. At one time tennis was a game of grace. Now it has become a game of big serves and lot of power. Long practice is required which can fatigue an elderly person. All the time there has to be good control while twisting to avoid back from being injured or sprained. If this precaution is well taken then twisting sports are good. They help to loosen stiff muscles and ligaments and help increase mobility.

Ergonomics:

This word is used more frequently today. In its most basic term ergonomics means trying to fit the job to the person rather than fitting the person to the job. For example most of our chairs are meant for average sized persons. When this chair is given to an individual, one has to find if he can really sit comfortably in the chair or not. Ergonomics are well utilised today while making seats of the car. But if a given woman is short she may have to draw the seat nearer to reach the pedals only to notice that the steering wheel is too close to her chest. In short, recognition of human individuality at work is ergonomics. Ergonomics play an important role in maintaining spine alignment and reducing the fatigue experienced in the back at the end of the day. Whether one is sitting, standing or walking, ergonomics can be applied to everyone at home, during travel and at work. Solutions do not always involve costly changes. One has not to rebuild the wall cabinet if it is too high. A step stool can do the trick.

PART - IV

ESSENTIAL PRESENTING FEATURES OF BACKPAIN AND SCIATICA

PRESENTATION OF BACKPAIN

SYMPTOMS:

THE common symptoms of backpain are backache or pain in the back and stiffness. The pain is felt most at the time of injury and is described as stabbing in the back. It is at times excruciating and is aggravated by coughing and sneezing. The pain due to sprain is usually not in the cantre but on one side away from midline.

The pain of prolapsed lumbar intervertebral disc starts in the midline and spreads to one side. Very rarely the pain is felt on both sides of the midline. When back pain due to herniated lumbar intervertebral disc becomes chronic, usually the midline pain disappears and only the lateral component of the pain remains as residual pain and is usually felt in the sacro-iliac joint or in the buttock. The intensity of pain remains the same on the second and third day and then it starts becoming less.

Besides sneezing and coughing the pain also becomes worse with twisting movements when you try to turn on one side in bed. Forward bending and sitting appears impossible and the patient sticks to bed in one position. The pain is extremely unpleasant and the patient is terribly worried that if he does any abnormal movements he might get pain. A soft bed promotes twisting movements and hence the rationale of providing hard bed for the backache patients so that on a hard surface he can turn on one side as one piece without twisting.

Stiffness:

By next day the back feels stiff. One gets a feeling that the back has turned into a log of wood. This feeling is experienced in the morning. It improves slightly as the day progresses but again stiffness worsens by late afternoon. Spinal movements are restricted. The stiffness in the back lasts for at least two weeks and acute pain can last from days to weeks depending on the severity of the injury. Once the acute episode has passed one is left with a dull ache localised to the lumbosacral region.

Sciatica:

Along with back pain if there is associated herniated lumbar intervertebral disc and there is pressure on the nerve, then there will be additional symptoms. Common symptom is sciatic pain or pain along the sciatic nerve in the limb. Since the disc prolapse is most common in the lowest two intervertebral discs, from the pattern of pain in the leg it is possible to postulate as to which disc has prolapsed. The sciatic pain of 4th lumbar disc prolapse migrates from the back of the thigh straight to the big toe and pain from prolapse of 5th lumbar disc migrates up to the ankle joint.

If the disc prolapse is central and there is evidence of lumbar canal stenosis then pain is felt in both calf muscles on standing and walking and is relieved on lying down. True sciatic pain in one leg is not always relieved on lying down.

Associated Symptoms:

Along with pain in the back and in the legs there are other associated symptoms such as :

    A : Numbness in the legs and feet.
    B : Shooting pain in the buttocks.
    C : Weakness in the feet and ankle joint.
    D : At times weakness in the quadriceps muscles of the thigh.
    E : Awkwardness in walking.
    F : Bladder disturbances in certain cases.

Usually, there is difficulty in passing urine and the bladder feels distended. The numbness and weakness is felt in the same leg with pain. Presence of weakness and difficulty in passing urine are more sinister symptoms. They should not be treated with home medicines and/or neglected. The specialist spinal surgeon should be consulted immediately. If the symptoms are not very severe, the doctor himself may suggest conservative treatment for you. The doctor will advise hospitalisation if conservative treatment has failed or the symptoms, in the opinion of the doctor, are severe enough to need further tests and possible surgery.

A PATIENT OF PROLAPSED DISC IN THE HOUSE:

A patient of prolapsed disc can easily be spotted in the crowd.

He lies crouched up in bed. Stretching legs is uncomfortable.

He keeps his legs bent at knee and hip joints.

He walks stiff like a robot, with short steps.

To look behind he has to turn as a whole like a log of wood.

He is bent on one side with drooping of shoulder and indrawing of abdomen.

He cannot bend forwards to brush his teeth.

He looks ill and apprehensive.

During the acute phase he remains uncooperative during changing clothes, cleaning, etc.

If symptoms last long, he becomes irritable and depressed.

Viewed from the back, the spine is twisted.

Muscles of the spine are prominent and buttocks loose their shape from weakness and wasting.

PART - V

GUIDELINES FOR MANAGEMENT

* HOME REMEDIES
* CONSULTATIONS
* SURGERY
* FITNESS

PART - V

ONCE YOU HAVE BACKPAIN

MANAGEMENT:

WITH an attack of backpain it is important first to consult the doctor before any treatment is started. The treatment will depend on the cause of the symptoms. The treatment of prolapsed disc syndrome is different from the treatment of a simple backsprain. Backpain may be due to other causes as described above. The condition must be first properly diagnosed, before treatment is begun.

Investigations:

In a given case of backsprain or prolapsed lumbar intervertebral disc one does not require too many investigations. The set of investigations required are simple and straightforward.

Plain X-rays of the Lumbar Spine:

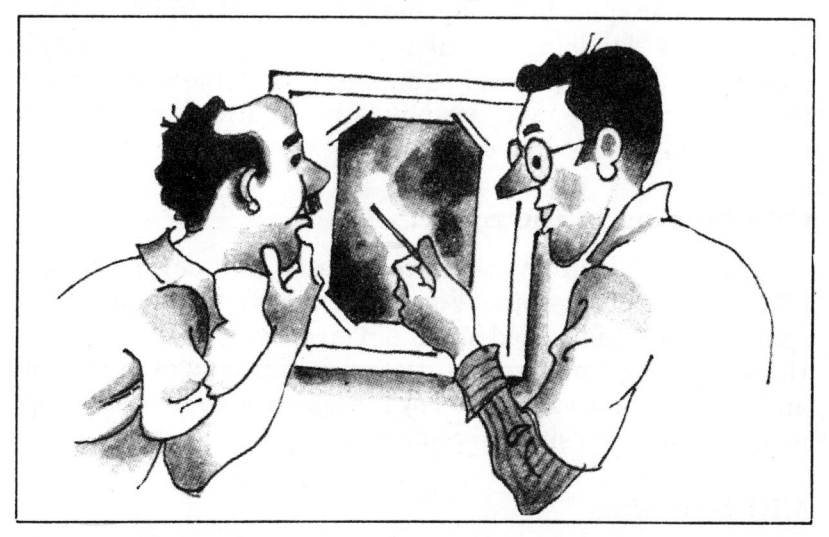

Fig. 12: A doctor will explain to you on your X rays the cause of backache and sciatica.

These are done in two planes (Antero Posterior 'AP' and Lateral 'Lat'.) Sometimes two more X-rays are done in oblique positions. The X-rays are done on an empty stomach in the morning after a dose of purgative the previous night so that all the gas in the bowels is expelled. These X-rays are not exactly useful for the diagnosis of a prolapsed disc. The X-rays may give indirect hint of a prolapsed disc if the disc space is reduced due to degeneration in the intervertebral disc. If the spine is twisted or rotated to one side (list of the spine or scoliotic spine) it may suggest the presence of underlying disc. It also rules out the presence of other abnormalities like spondylolysis or spondylolisthesis or fracture of the spine. Plain X-rays are done more to exclude other pathological conditions than to diagnose a prolapsed disc.

Myelography:

This investigation was very much in vogue before the advent of CT Scans and MRI Scanning of the lumbar spine. Myelogram is a good investigation and gives accurate diagnosis of a prolapsed disc. However, it is rather invasive in the sense that contrast dye is to be injected in the subarachnoid space of the lumbar spine by giving an injection in the spine or what is known as "by doing a lumbar puncture". Not many people like it. The thought of taking an injection in the spine scares them away. Hence myelography is not routinely carried out today in big cities like Bombay.

CT Scanning of the Spine:

After myelography the investigation that developed was CT Scanning of the spine. For some time CT Scanning on the spine was routinely used and it did give accurate information. However it could not produce reconstruction images in sagittal and coronal planes as desired by the spinal surgeons, although it was a non-invasive procedure.

MRI Scanning:

With the advent of MRI Scanning the CT Scan fell behind

in the imaging of lumbar spine. Today most lumbar spines are investigated with the help of MRI Scanning. It gives accurate information about the size, shape and location of the prolapsed disc. It also gives information about the size of the bony canal and any other abnormalities if present. The investigation is non-invasive and can be done at any time of the day. It can even be done in a patient with acute pain if the patient can lie in one position for a few minutes.

Today just two investigations, namely plain X-rays of the spine and MRI Scanning are enough to arrive at conclusion regarding diagnosis of the cause of pain in a given patient with backache and sciatica.

HOME REMEDIES FOR BACKACHE:

Most of the times if one gets an attack of backpain which is more often a sprain it helps to keep the head cool and take two aspirins. At the beginning of this century only remedies available for relief of pain were Aspirin. Salsaparila and hot water springs containing sulphur. Times have changed and lot of other analgesic and anti-inflammatory agents are now available.

In an acute attack of backpain late in the evening it helps just to take a Combiflam tablet. Understandably in an acute attack this advice may not seem reasonable. The patient's expectations are much more and he wishes to have an urgent appointment with the doctor. Hard it may sound to believe but more often two Combiflam tablets do the trick. It does not help to panic. Unless of course if the patient looses control over his bowels or bladder then it is a serious problem and one need to consult the doctor immediately and perhaps he will need emergency hospitalisation.

If the backpain does not get better with rest and anti-inflammatory drugs within three days then one must seek the appointment of a specialist spinal surgeon. Going to the doctor makes sense. Following examination he is in a position to make out if the patient has developed prolapsed intervertebral disc and if there is pressure on the nerves.

SERIOUS CONSEQUENCES:
MUST SEE A DOCTOR:

Most backpains start feeling better within a day or two. But if the pain gets worse then one must consult a doctor. As said earlier difficulty in passing urine or opening bowels is a strong indication to consult a specialist immediately. Most of the times, in these cases the nerves are affected and require urgent attention of the doctor.

Foot drop: Dragging a foot because the muscles have become weak or paralysed is a serious neurological problem such as compression of the nerve by prolapsed disc. If this symptom is ignored it can leave one permanently dragging his foot.

TAKE REST:

First basic concept of acute backsprain is to stop doing whatever activity one is engaged with and take rest so that the part which is sprained is not further insulted. It is difficult at times to believe but a golfer having hurt his back at the second hole will continue to play till the last hole. This is not correct.

The part which is sprained must be immediately rested. For years, bed rest has been a common treatment for backsprains.

In the past it was not unusual for the doctor to instruct the patient to take rest for weeks and even months. Even today it is common for this practice being followed in many places. I do not agree with this practice. Research has shown that prolonged bed rest is in fact more harmful. Muscles start wasting, capsules of the joints start contracting and bones loose their calcium.

When bed rest and anti-inflammatory drugs do not help within a reasonable period of maximum one week, a specialist should be consulted.

Please remember the following instructions to get maximum out of your bed rest.
1. Relax the spine completely.
2. Do not lie face down.
3. Lie on your back with a pillow under the knee.
4. Lie on the side with a pillow between the knees.
5. Distract your mind from the pain. Watch television, read light humorous stories; listen to soothing music.

DRUGS:

Most of the times the cause of backpain as an acute episode with or without sciatica can be attributed to irritated muscles, stretched ligaments, inflamed capsule of the facet joints, a swollen disc or stretched nerve root. In these circumstances drugs which prevent or halt inflammation are effective. As said above, Ibuprofen is the best among all the anti-inflammatory drugs available today. Aspirin because it causes gastric irritation is not used. Ibuprofen in doses of 400 mg. three times a day along with paracetamol (Combiflam) not only reduces inflammation but helps to reduce pain and other symptoms usually associated with inflammation. Hence the best medicine for home use today is Combiflam which is a combination of 400 mg. of Ibuprofen and 325 mg. of paracetamol.

Combiflam should be immediately taken after injury for better relief. But it should not be taken on an empty stomach.

Anti-inflammatory drugs should not be taken on an empty stomach. It causes gastric irritation. They should be taken after a meal or breakfast. Combiflam three times a day is adequate. Do not try to overdose. Drugs taken in higher doses have side effects which are not good for the body.

Drugs such as diazepam help to relax the muscles and calm the nerves. Five mg. three times a day in the initial stages and then only one tablet at bedtime is adequate. Chymōlripsin helps if there is bruise in the muscles and antacids help to prevent gastric irritation.

Fomentation: (Ice or Heating Pad):

Sports principles is followed. During the first forty eight hours ice should be applied. It prevents swelling and is soothing. After 48 hours heating pad increases blood circulation in the deeper tissue. This helps to relax the muscles. Later when you visit the physiotherapy center the heating pad can be replaced with short wave diathermy. Infra red lamp does not penetrate deeper into the tissues and is not quite effective. Whatever heat one uses it should not be done excessively or without little care to avoid burning the skin.

Massage:

Gentle massage helps to loosen the tight muscles in spasm. But this should not be used during the first 48 hours when there is acute inflammation. It should be used after the acute inflammation and swelling has subsided. Massage has additional benefit. The anxiety of the patient is relieved along with the relief in pain. Gentle massage after a couple of days should be encouraged. Massage should be done with fingers without using any oil. In fact fingers can be replaced with massagers and vibrators readily available in the market.

Traction and Bed Rest:

Traction is a form of physical therapy. More than anything else it restricts the patient to the bed and assures unwanted

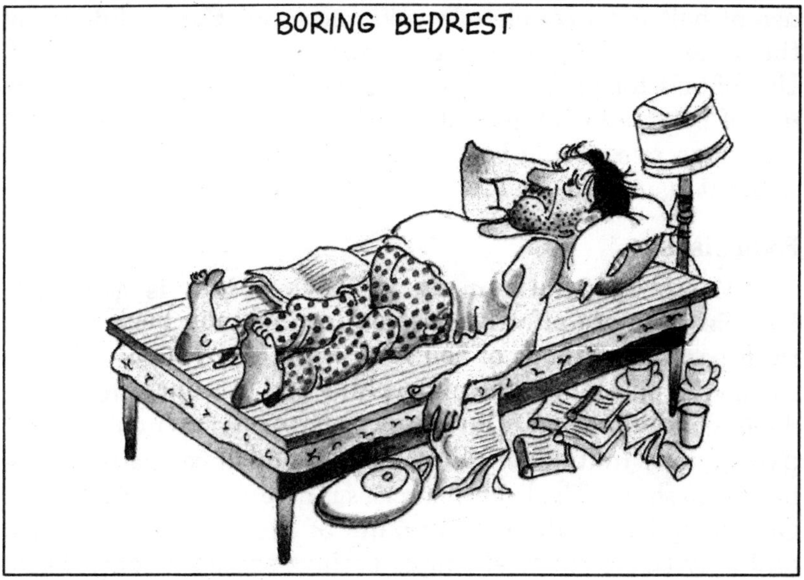

Fig. 13: Bed rest is boring and is like solitary confinement. Not many people like it.

bed rest to allow the back to heal. The weight should not be too much. The traction on the back should be gentle. It is presumed that stretching may relieve the pressure on the nerve and thus help to relieve pain. It can be given continuously or intermittently say twice a day. However continuous traction for prolonged periods does not conform to the sport principle of early activity. If it restricts the patient to bed continuously over prolonged periods say three weeks it should not be encouraged. Traction should not be forced on the patient. If found uncomfortable it should be immediately removed. Continuous bed rest with or without traction is not popular among patients.

Lumbosacral Belt:

The idea of belt is to prevent too much movement during the painful phase. After an episode of backache when one moves about and goes to work lumbosacral belt gives confidence to the patient by restricting excessive movements. After surgery use of belt for a couple of weeks increases the confidence of the patient to do his exercises regularly and with enthusiasm. Use of belt for prolonged periods should be discouraged. The use of belt and exercises should be so well harmonised that very soon one should be able to walk freely with confidence without using the belt.

Exercises:

Most beneficial remedy for back sprain is exercises. Exercise is more effective in treating common back sprains than passive methods of bed rest. Exercise by itself releases the body's painkillers the endorphins and it reduces too much dependence on drugs. During recovery exercise must become part of daily routine for relieving pain and once again getting back into shape. The list of exercises is given in the supplement. One should carefully do minimum of exercises to start with and may be for the first couple of days should do only warm up exercises. Restoration of lordosis or natural curve of the spine, lessen stiffness and increase flexibility after backpain is the purpose of the exercises. Once the relief from pain is achieved one can start back strengthening exercises.

The best exercise to start with is press up exercise and it can be done several times in a day. Another exercise that helps at this stage is walking. The purpose of exercise is to improve circulations. Extra blood supply helps the tissues to heal faster. The goal is to pump warm oxygen filled blood into the injured tissues and to do this one has to sweat a bit for good results. But it will need time, patience and practice before you can reach this stage after injury. Fresh oxygen and increased tissue temperature helps to relax the muscles in spasm.

Do not be Anxious:

Biofeedback in simple terms means the therapy of suggestion which is found to be very effective specially with spastic hemiplegics. Medical evidence suggests that depression and anxiety can have bad effects on the body including back pain. Our natural reaction to pain is to tense the muscles to protect the painful part. Tensed muscles increase the pain which in turn increase anxiety. One can get around this problem by learning relaxation techniques. One must learn to relax by one's own suggestions (auto-suggestion) and if this is not possible then one should adopt guided suggestions from an instructor but auto-suggestions is the best therapy. Create a beautiful scene in front of your eyes and virtually get lost into it. Even if one is lost into the scene for ten minutes, it is beneficial to relieve anxiety.

Sexual Functions:

Once there is pain sexual functions take a back seat. Sexual function is a recreation. One cannot utilise it during acute pain. During this period one should find recreation in watching television or music or later playing cards. Sex as recreation could be extremely important during recovery phase. Pain is the greatest factor limiting sex. A patient in pain is always worried that sex may bring the attack again. The best way to convince one self is to maintain activity during recovery phase and thus increase confidence. For a person recovering from backpain sex is safe as long as the activity causes minimal pain.

Other Forms of Treatment:

Many doctors give steroid injections into the facet joints or in the epidural space combined with anaesthetic agent. It does relieve pain albeit temporarily. It cannot give long lasting relief. Same is the story of chiropractitioners, osteopaths and manipulators. In chronic degenerative spine they do produce relief which is gratifying even temporarily but they should know their limitations. There are innumerable examples where a back with large prolapsed disc was manipulated and patient developed neurological complications. It would be always prudent first to consult a specialist and then undergo manipulation if one so desires.

Hospitalisation:

If the backpain and sciatica have not settled with conservative treatment and if the doctor is satisfied that one is suffering from a large prolapsed disc then he will advise surgery. With the advance in spinal surgery the operation for prolapsed lumbar intervertebral disc has become simple for the patient with less and less time to be spent in the hospital. If one is suffering from pure prolapsed disc causing pain in one of the legs than surgery can be done with microscope known as microlumbar discectomy. It has least morbidity and the patient can virtually be discharged from the hospital within 24 hours.

Surgery:

If one is scheduled for surgery then depending on age certain tests like examination of blood, X-ray of the chest, cardiogram, etc. are carried out to decide the patient's suitability to undergo general anaesthesia. The day prior to the operation the anaesthetist will check the patient and see that one is not allergic to any drugs. Light supper is given in the evening before surgery and a sleeping tablet to pass a comfortable night.

Usually an enema is given early in the morning and an hour before operation the patient is given a sedative dose of medicine.

The operation is carried out under general anaesthesia and one does not come to know anything about it. Next thing the patient finds himself lying comfortably in his own bed in the room.

If microlumbar discectomy has been done then patient is allowed to get out of bed on the same day in the evening to walk upto the toilet.

Certain amount of pain is expected during the first 48 hours but a tablet of painkiller makes life comfortable. Light diet may be given in the evening of the operation.

Activity:

If one has undergone microlumbar discectomy then one is allowed to move about freely on the next day and is even discharged home. However if one has undergone laminectomy then the patient is restricted to bed for at least three days and then allowed to get out of bed gradually and is discharged home on the sixth day.

When one feels comfortable, the exercises on the back are started gradually and slowly not to hurt the back. The exercises can be increased as the confidence of the patient mounts higher. This is a better way rather than rushing through the exercises, hurting the back and realising a setback in the activity programme.

After Discharge:

Having gone home do not try to do too much. Determine the level of activity depending on the feeling of tiredness. If one feels tired easily it is a warning to slow down. It is advisable after back surgery not to do heavy work or lift heavy loads for two months.

Walking may seem tiring but starting with a short walk in the morning if one increases the distance gradually then walking is the best activity after surgery on the back. Regular exercise will bring back full strength in the spinal muscles and once this is achieved one will forget that he has undergone surgery on the back. The scar is usually seen as a thin line which is not more than one inch long in case microlumbar discectomy has been done.

Given oneself a little time say maximum three months, there are no restrictions on the usual activity of the person after lumbar disc surgery.

Once a disc has been removed usually that disc does not prolapse again. If any time in future there is recurrence of symptoms usually the symptoms are due to a disc higher up than the one operated upon.

Hundreds of thousand of operations are being carried out on the back every year round the world. If one requires surgery it should be done expeditiously and be pleased with the results.

Whether the therapy was conservative or surgical there is every reason to expect that the daily life will be significantly improved as a result of having undergone proper treatment and proper rehabilitation for a given case of prolapsed lumbar intervertebral disc or a simple backsprain.

SUPPLEMENT:

EXERCISES TO KEEP THE BACK AND THE BODY HEALTHY

(TO BE CARRIED OUT AT HOME)

KEEP YOUR BACK IN SHAPE

THIS supplement concentrates on day-to-day practical tips so that back can be kept in shape. The set of choice exercises are fully illustrated and explained. Followed regularly they will help prevent backpain and keep the back and the body in shape. Rehabilitation after an attack of backpain becomes easy. Maintaining a regular exercise programme is the best way to prevent back from attacks of sprains and pains.

PURPOSE OF THE EXERCISE PROGRAMME:

A set of exercises done regularly has following advantages:

1. Extensor muscles at the back of the spine are the main weight lifters of the spine. They are strengthened by the exercises.

2. The abdominal muscles are most important to keep the spine in proper alignment. Most of the times the abdominal muscles are weak and flabby. Strengthening these muscles helps to keep the spine in proper alignment.

3. Other muscles of the trunk are toned and stabilised so that the spine gets added power and strength.

4. The muscles of the leg share with the muscles of spine the burden of lifting the weight. In fact, the quadriceps muscles of the thigh is the horsepower of the body. By doing exercise regularly these muscles are strengthened and they then contribute to the strength of the spine.

5. Agility, flexibility and stretchability of the spine is improved with exercises and the spine looks younger with advancing age. You will feel proud to realise this.

GENERAL INSTRUCTIONS BEFORE DOING EXERCISES:

1. The exercises must be done on a hard floor. The open ground which is good for jogging is not good for exercises.

2. To start with, do all the exercises five times each. Increase the number as the strength in the muscles increases. One should not feel tired.

3. Be well relaxed and at ease. Do not fit the exercise programme in ten minutes that you have to spare before leaving for the airport. Exercises can be done at any time provided the stomach is not full after a heavy meal.

4. Use as little clothing as is possible. The clothes in the exercises as illustrated here are tightly fitting for the purpose of demonstration. It is preferable to use loose clothing.

5. Do not hold breath. Keep breathing rhythmically while doing exercises. This requires a little practice. The tendency generally is to hold the breath. Holding breath may lead to bad effects.

6. If an exercise causes pain, abandon it. If a particular exercise causes pain repeatedly, then consult the doctor.

7. Preferably do the exercises in front of the mirror if you have one. There is always the emotional satisfaction of achievement.

8. Doing exercises in company has added advantages although not essential. Many times backache is psychosomatic and tension myositis is one example. At

times exercise programme is a function of suggestion. Group therapy is advantageous. Therapeutic exercises are today established as an important aspect of treatment of backpain.

YOU DO NOT REQUIRE TOO MUCH EQUIPMENT:

An effective home exercise programme as illustrated here requires practically nothing. Whatever equipment is required is already available at home.

Most important requirement is motivation and your determination. Starting is easy. To continue with the exercise requires determination. Once this is achieved then exercise programme becomes as simple as brushing teeth in the morning.

EXERCISES AFTER SURGERY ON THE BACK:

Exercises are extremely important after surgery on the back. Following surgery stiffness is usually produced in the back due to operative adhesions. The set of home exercises are beneficial to increase the flexibility and increase the range of motion.

The exercises should be started as soon as it is possible after surgery. Crooked spine is generally seen in those suffering from backpain. This is known as postural aberration. These postural aberrations are effectively corrected by doing exercises.

WARM UP EXERCISES

WARM UP EXERCISES:

In theses exercises the muscles are stretched, the tendons are pulled and the joints are lubricated.

The cardio-pulmonary system is geared to produce the needed extra energy.

WARM UP EXERCISES :

Before doing the exercises the body must be prepared for it. The muscles should be lightly stretched, the tendons lightly pulled and the joints lubricated to prepare for the exercises. Similarly the cardio-pulmonary system i.e. the heart and the lungs must be warmed by activating them lightly to warn them of the oncoming activity in which they will have to work and co-ordinate to produce the required additional energy. This is done by a set of light exercises known as warm up exercises.

No pain should be felt during these exercises and one should feel the gradual stretch of the muscles and a sense of easing the body.

TYPE OF EXERCISES: Isometric versus Dynamic:

Exercises generally are of two types. In isometric exercises a specified portion of the body is held in one position against resistance for a given length of time. In dynamic exercises the part of the body is moving continuously in rhythm rather slowly. Both type of exercises are important for shaping the spine and in the set demonstrated here both these exercises are incorporated.

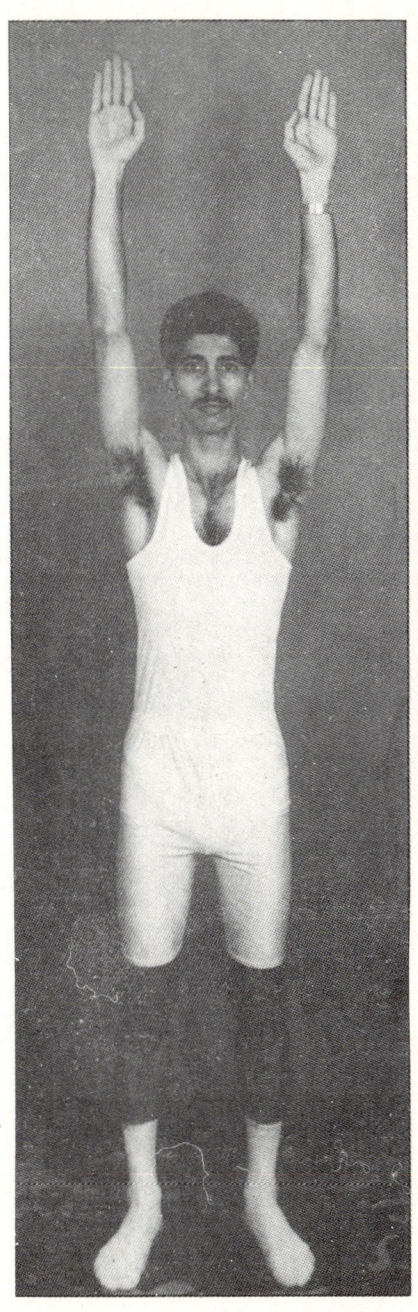

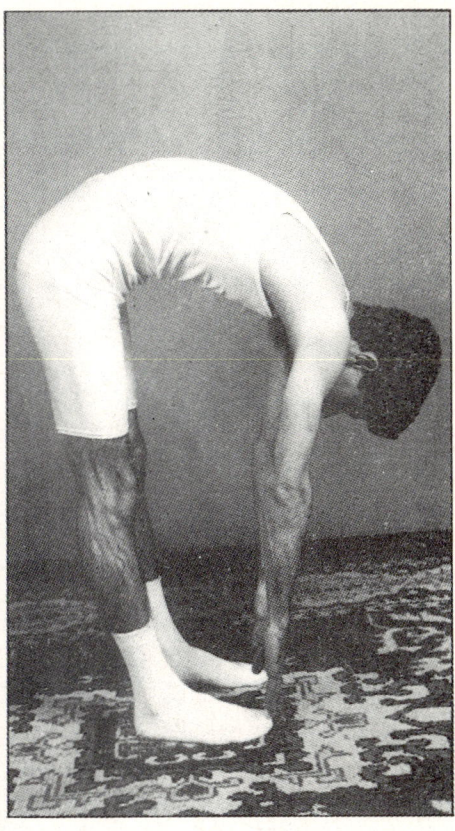

Stretching in Flexion:

Standing erect, the arms are raised and gradually brought down in a curvilinear fashion till one can (if possible) touch the toes. To start with, touching the toes may be difficult. Bend down as much as is possible. With the rhythm of the motion gradually straighten up and raise the arms. In a slow gliding rhythm repeat the exercise about twenty times.

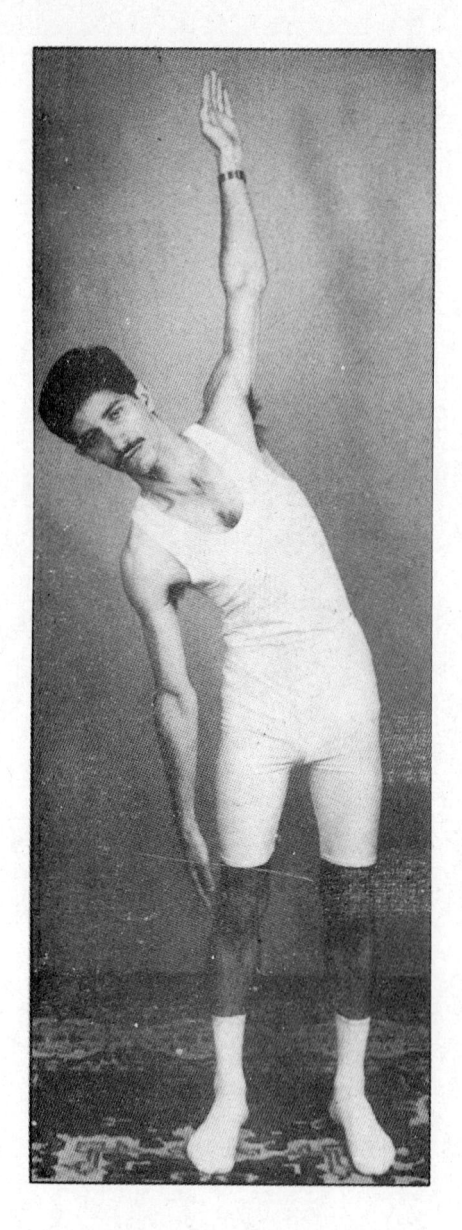

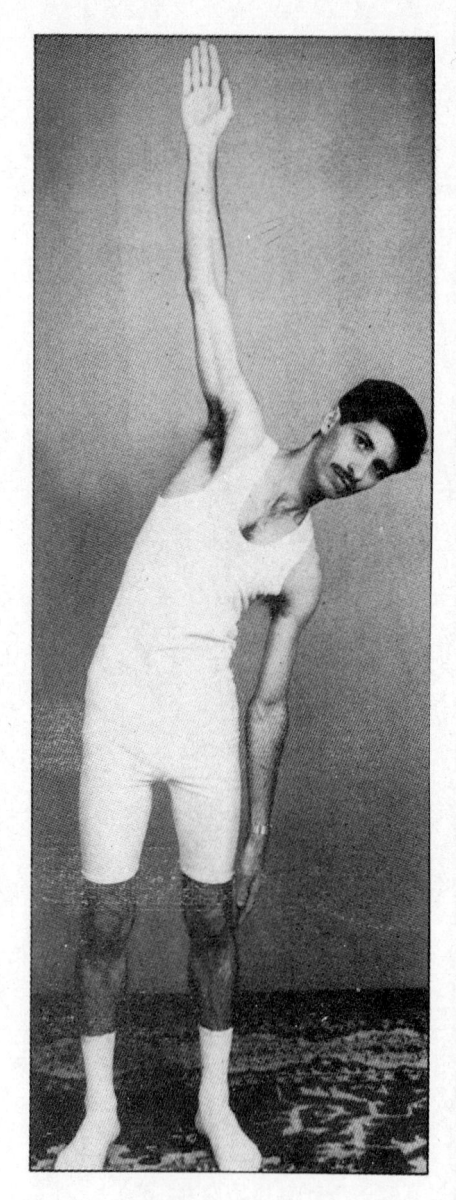

Lateral Stretching:

Hold both arms stretched on either side. Gradually bend on one side and then on the other side without twisting the body. Repeat the exercise twenty times while you are breathing regularly.

Stretching in Extension:

Hold the arms on the loins on either side and stand erect. Gradually stretch the body and the head to the back in a slow and sustained motion and then return back to the original position. People suffering from vertigo may find this exercise difficult. In that case this exercise should be omitted. Repeat the exercise ten times.

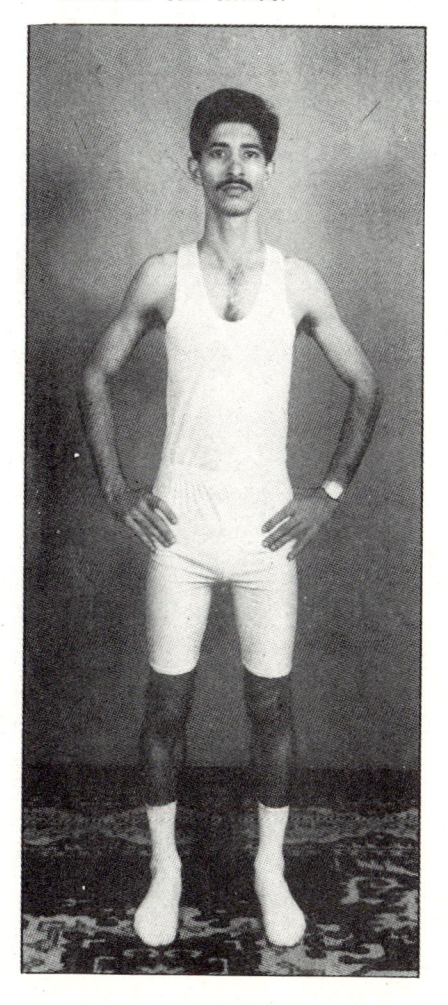

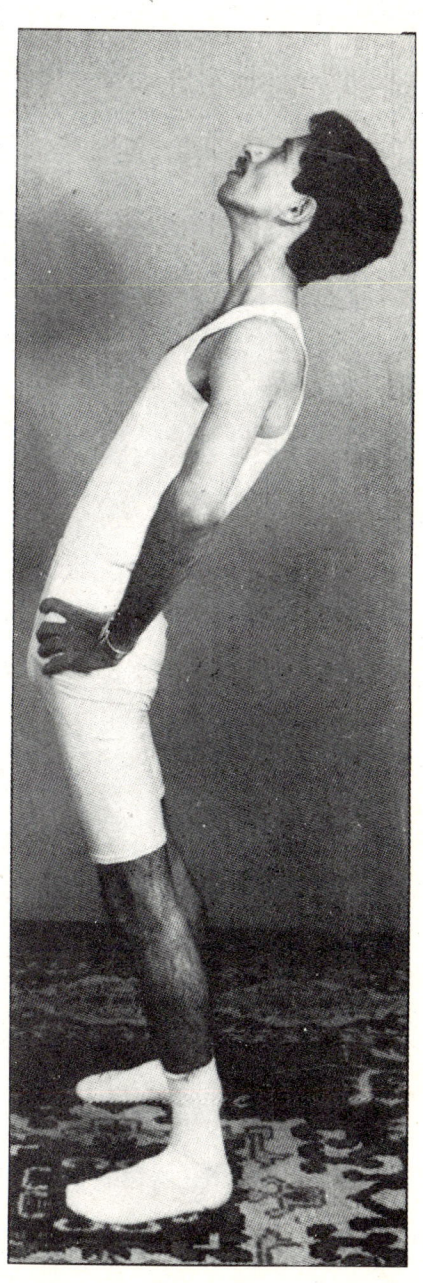

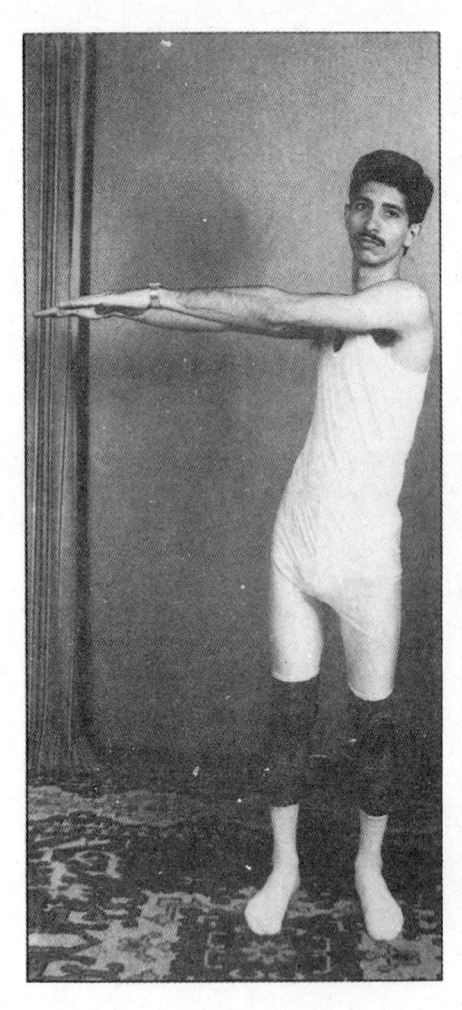

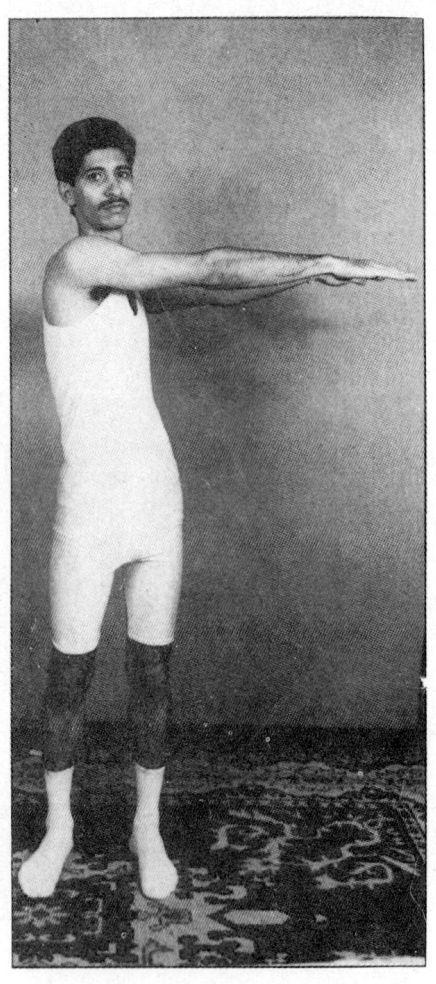

Rotational Stretching:

Hold both arms stretched in front of you and keep them parallel. First turn the arms to left side then come to the centre and turn the hands to the right side in one rhythmic motion. Repeat the exercise twenty times.

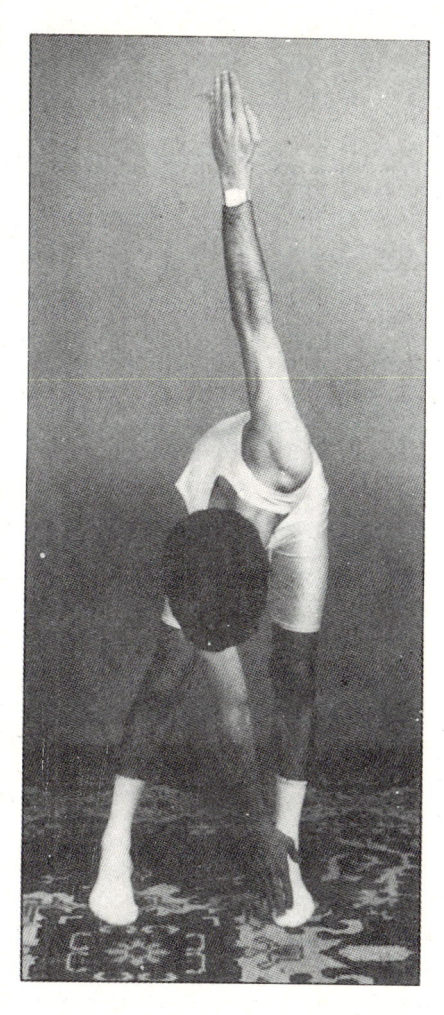

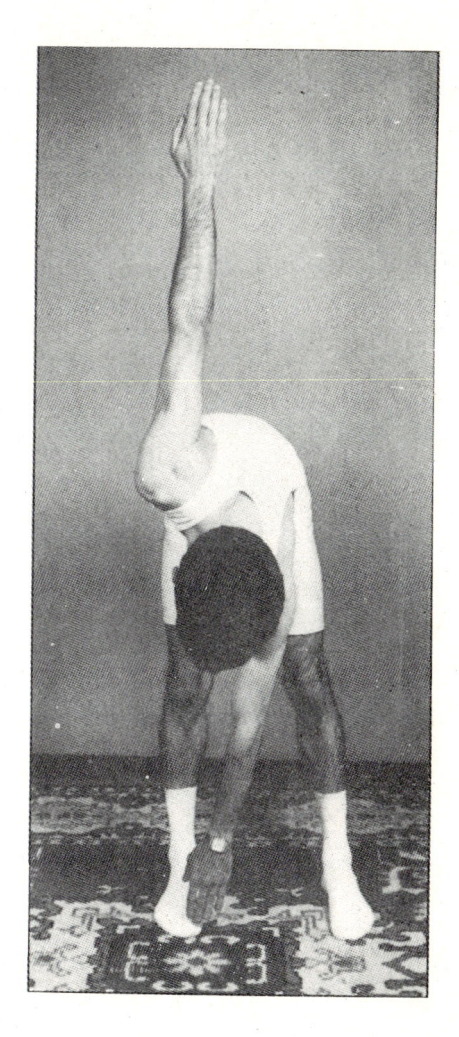

Stretching and Twisting:

Stand erect. Separate the two legs to a comfortable distance of one and half feet. Stretch both arms laterally. Without bending the knees or arms first touch the left great toe with right arm and then touch the right great toe with left arm. Repeat the exercise in rhythm ten times to start with.

Beginners and people with protruding belly will find this exercise difficult and in that case one should do whatever is possible without stretching oneself too much. It may lead to pain.

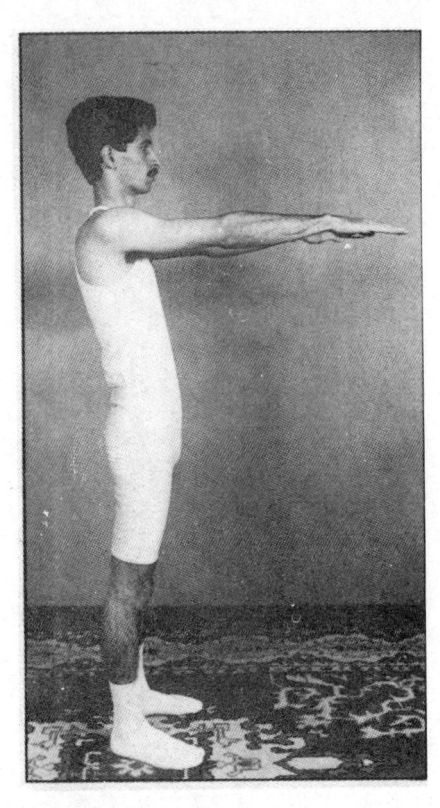

Sit ups:

Stand with arms stretched. Squat and straighten the hollow in the back. Return to standing position and repeat fifteen times.

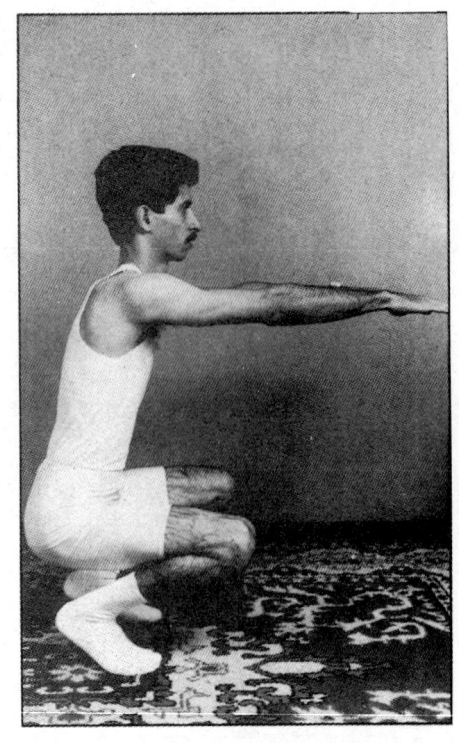

AT the end of this set of exercises the warm up and stretching is over. The body will start feeling warm and stretched and relaxed. The body is now ready for the main exercise. This warm up exercise automatically warms up the cardio pulmonary system to a point where it is now ready to supply the extra energy.

BACK STRENGTHENING EXERCISES

SET OF FLEXION EXERCISES

This set of exercises increases the postural stability. It is based on the assumption that there exists a postural instability due to inappropriate strength and flexibility of the abdominal and anterior spinal muscles particularly the strong Psoas muscles lying anteriorly on either side of the spine.

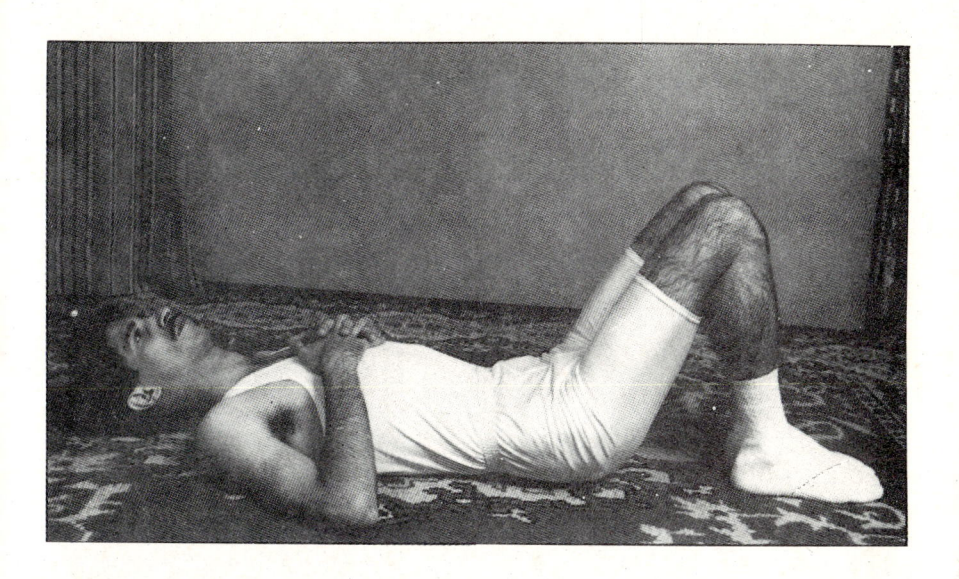

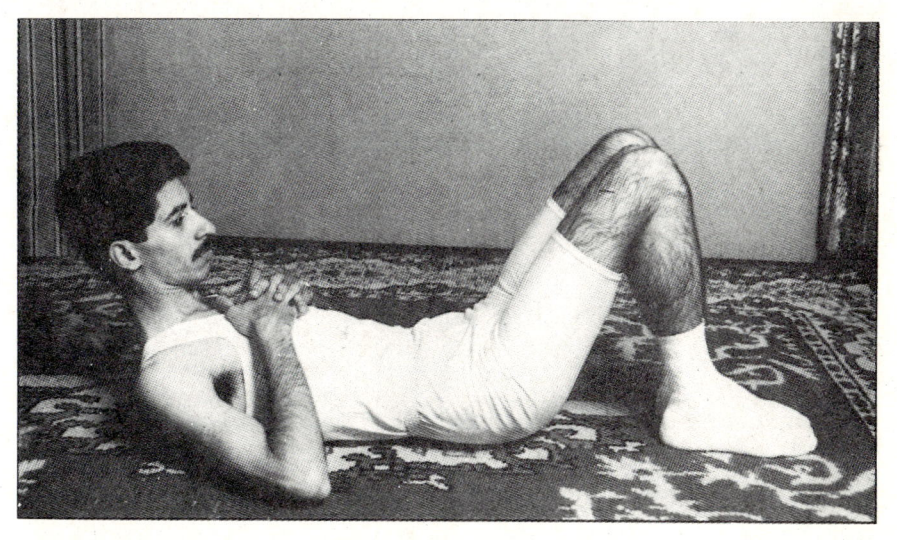

Abdominal Muscle Contraction:

Lie on the back with arms on chest and knees bent. Contract abdominal muscles towards spine by raising the head, hold for the count of ten and relax. Contract buttock muscles strongly and hold for the count of ten. Relax. Repeat the exercise fifteen times.

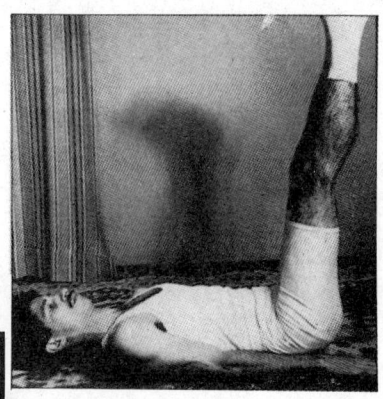

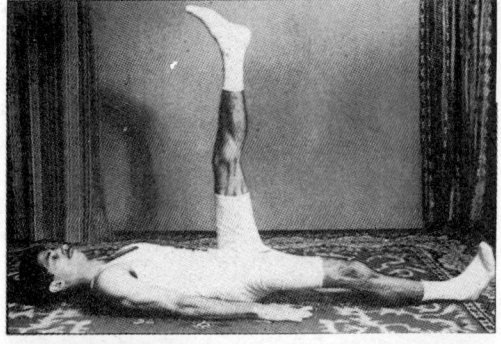

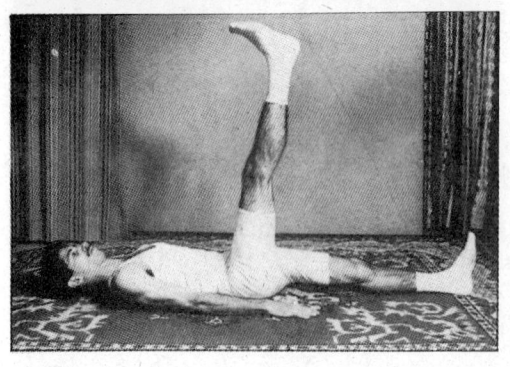

Straight Leg Raising:

Lie on back and hold the arms to the side. Lift one leg up without bending the knees and hold for the count of ten. Then bring it down slowly. Repeat the exercise with the other leg and repeat the performance ten times.

Simultaneous Both Legs Raising:

Lie flat on the floor with arms to the side and slowly in rhythm lift both legs up simultaneously to the point of comfort. Do not overstretch. If operated recently, this exercise may cause pain.

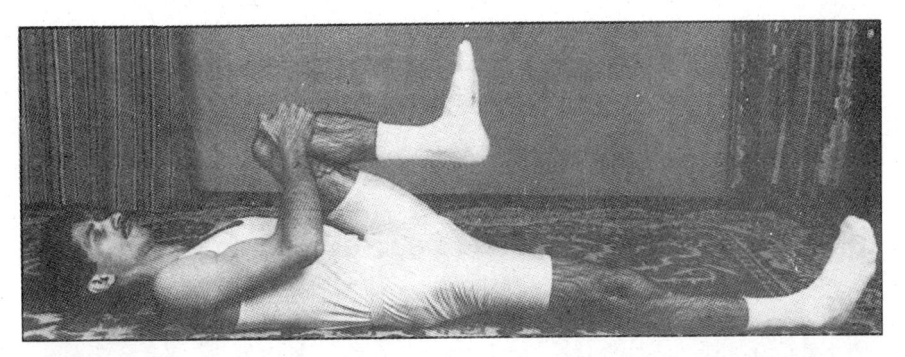

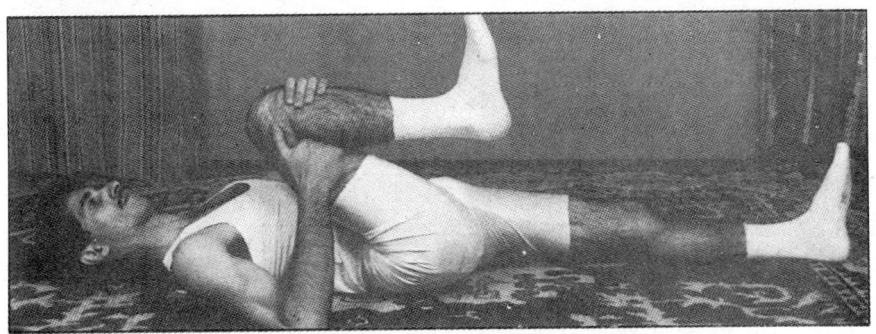

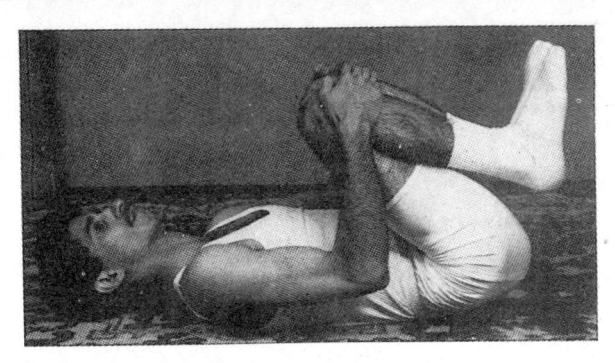

Single Knee to Chest Bend:

Lie flat on the back. With both arms lift one knee to chest and count ten. Then repeat the exercise with the other leg. Do this exercise fifteen times. This may bring pain in recently operated cases.

Double Knee to Chest Bend:

Lying flat on the back, lift both knees to chest and count ten. Do this exercise fifteen times.

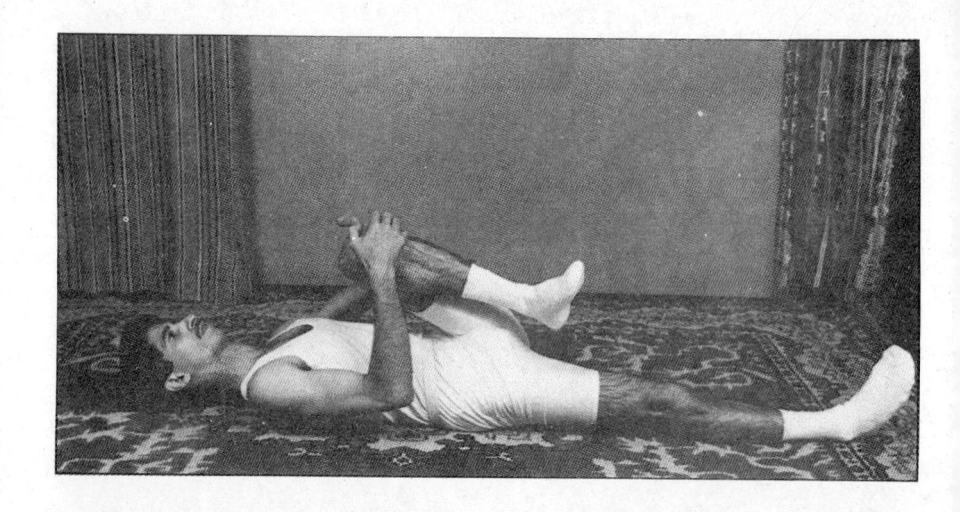

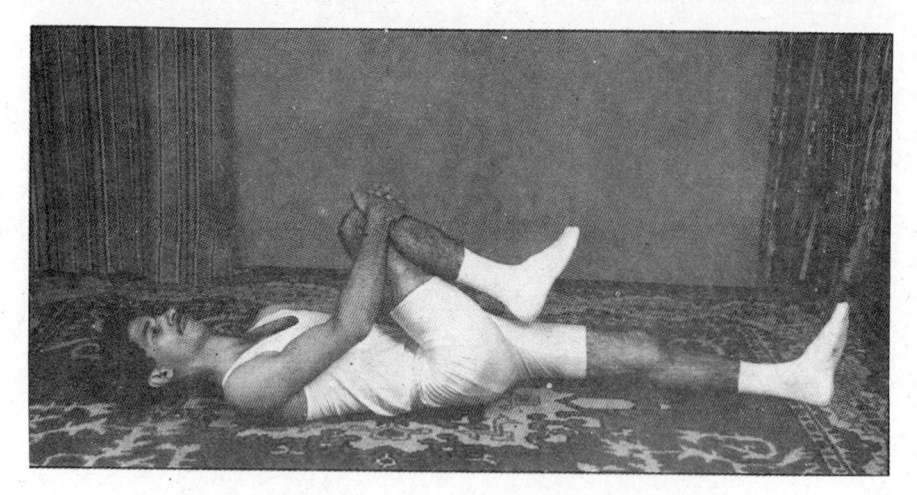

Oblique Knee Bend:

This exercise stretches the oblique muscles at the hip particularly the pyriformis muscle. Flex the leg with both arms at the knee. Then bend it obliquely as if to touch the opposite nipple. Hold for the count of ten. Relax and then repeat the exercise with the other leg. Repeat the exercise ten times.

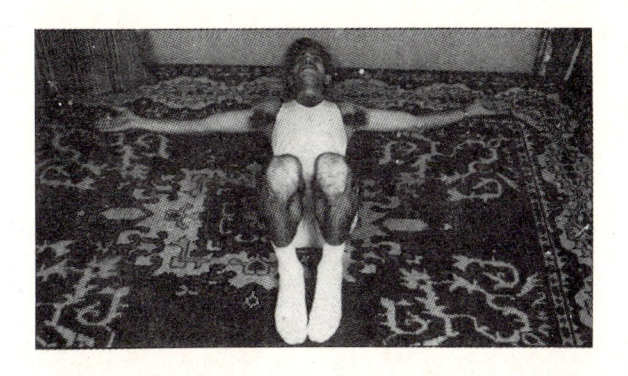

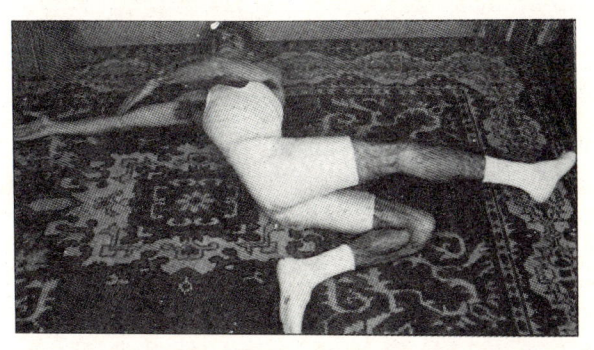

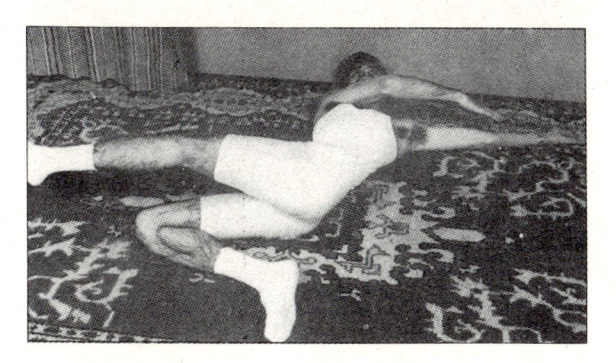

Advanced Lumbar Rotation:

Lie on back with knees bent and heels next to buttock. Stretch both arms on either side. Rotate the hip to the left side. Then stretch the right leg by extending it at the knee. Then rotate the left arm to the right side without moving the head. Keep the head in neutral position.

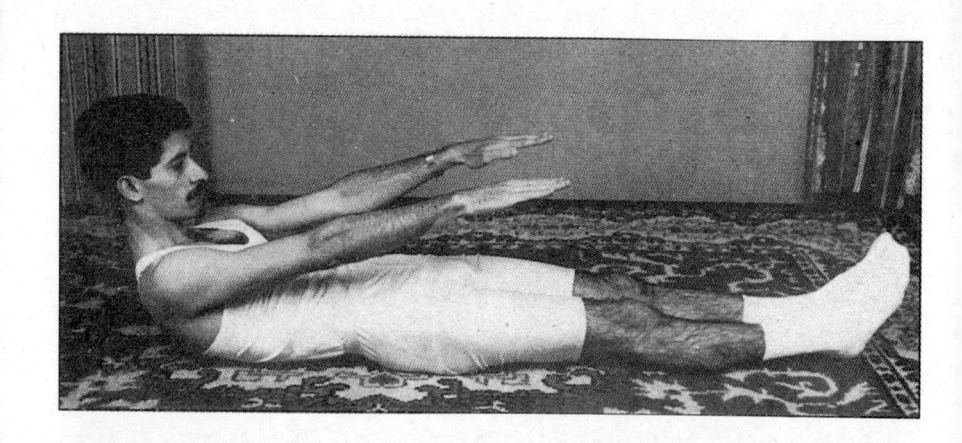

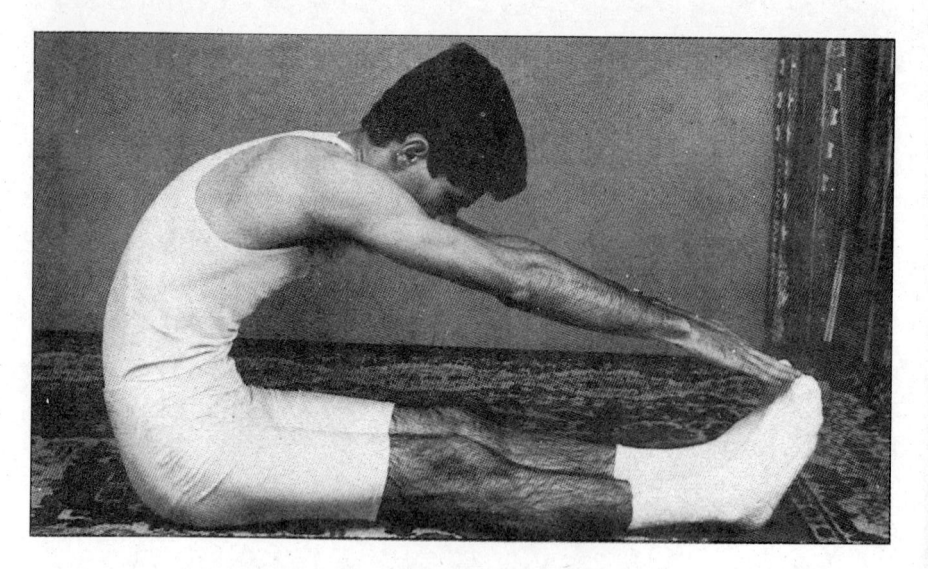

Abdominal Flexion with Spinal Stretch:

Lie on back with legs straight. Stretch both arms in front and sit up. Continue bending forwards till you can touch the toes with arms stretched and count ten. Repeat this difficult exercise five times.

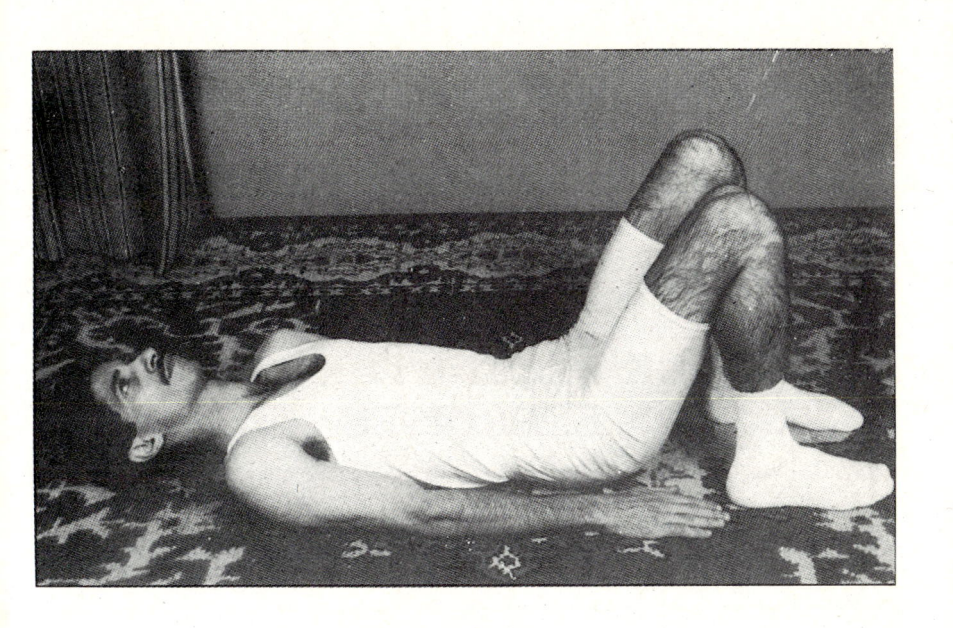

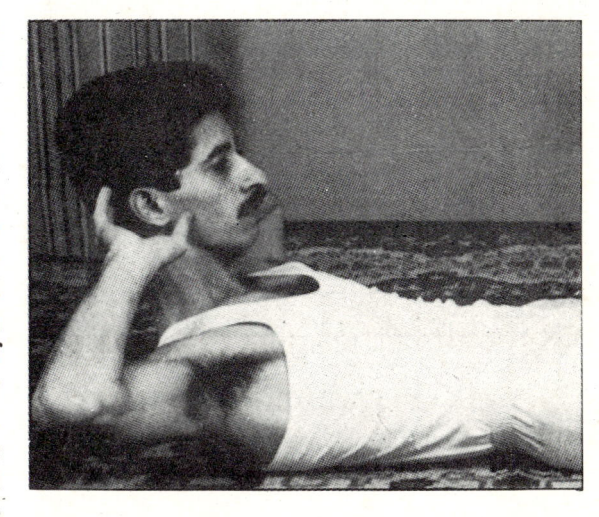

Advanced Aabdominal Flexion:

This is more difficult and must be done after one is well versed with other exercises. Lie on back with knees bent in a relaxed way and fingers of hands lightly touching the ears. Slowly raise up the head until shoulders leave the floor and then count ten and remember to breathe normally. Repeat this exercise five times.

BACK STRENGTHENING EXERCISES

SET OF EXTENSION EXERCISES

This set of exercise are meant to tone and build paraspinal muscles at the back of the spine lying on either side of the spinous processes. These muscles have great responsibility to make you look smart by holding the spine erect, pelvis tilted forward and chest broadly expanded.

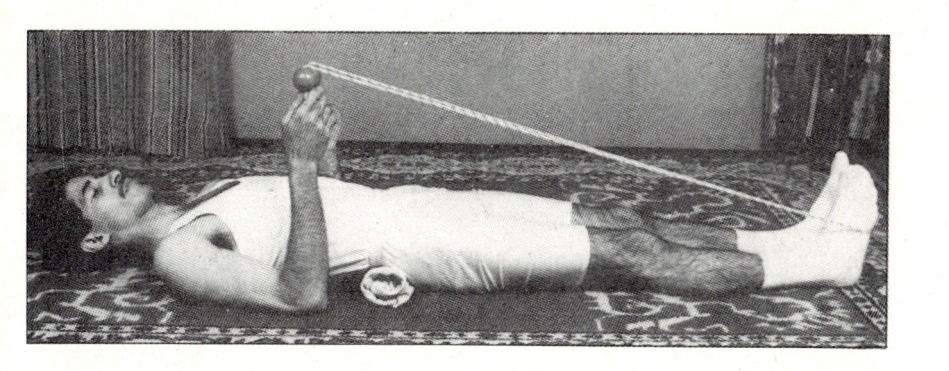

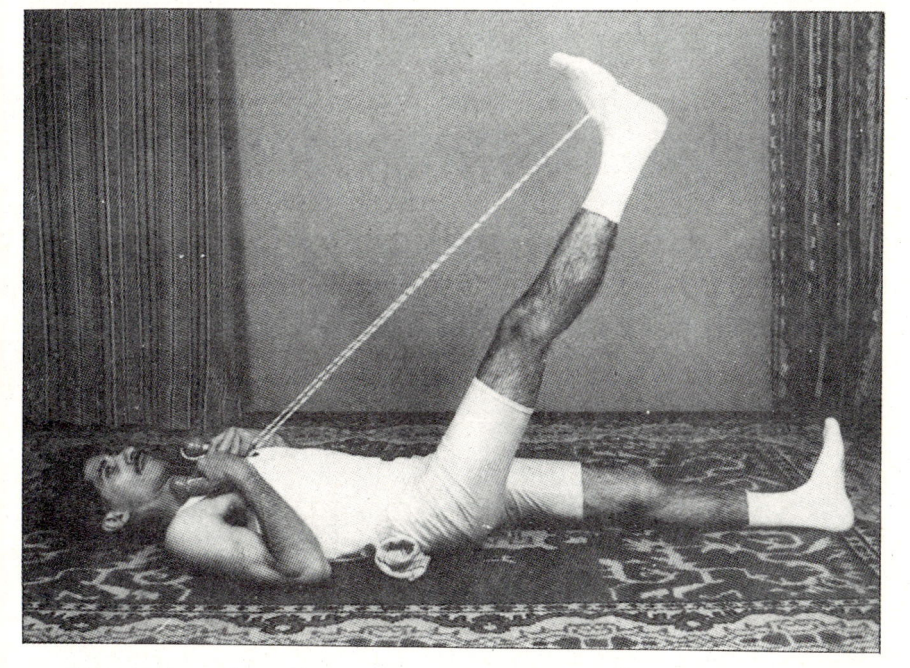

Hamstring Stretch:

This exercise helps to build up the muscles of thigh particularly the hamstring muscles.

Lie on back with a towel rolls up under the curve of the lumbar back. Place a rope around heel of right leg. With knee straight slowly lift right leg with rope towards chest and count ten. Then repeat with other leg. Do this exercise fifteen times.

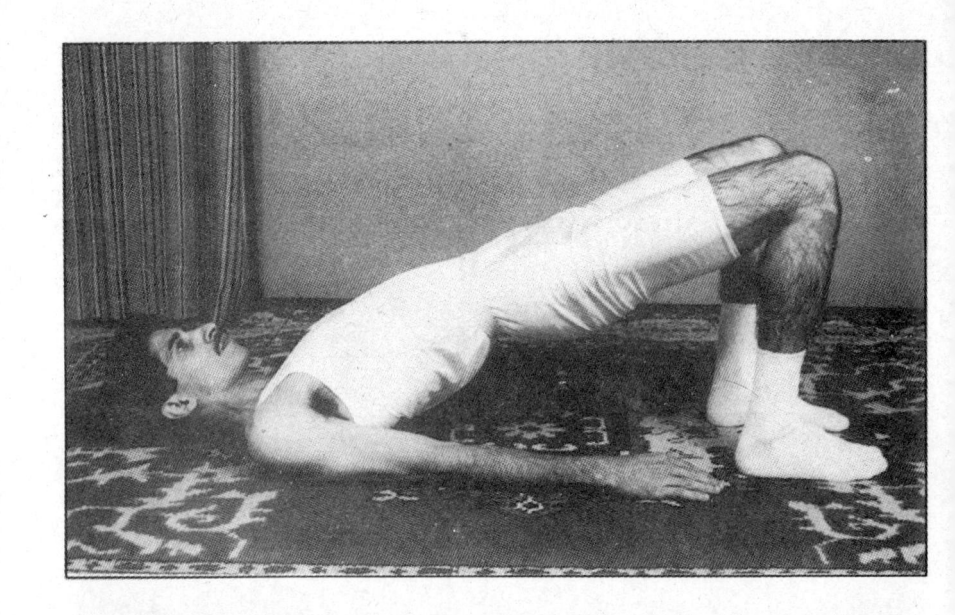

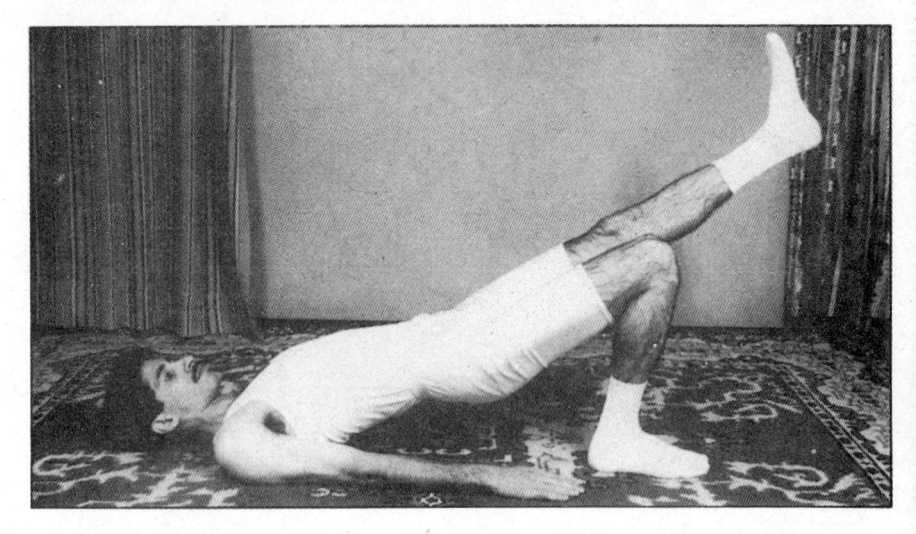

Bridging Exercise:

Lie on back with knees bent. Lift buttocks off the ground. Hold in that position. Extend the left leg at knee and count ten. Repeat the exercise with right leg. Repeat five times.

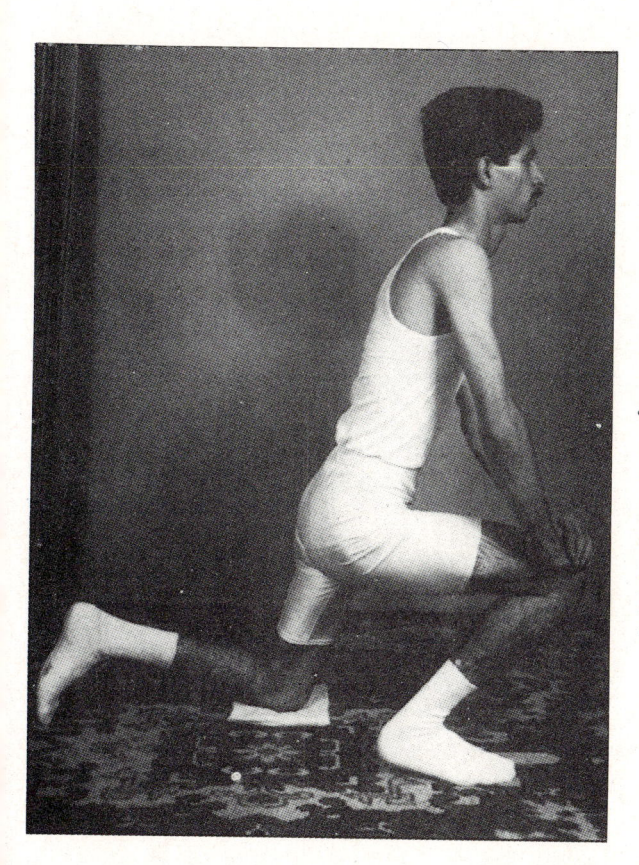

Hip Flexion and Stretch:

Place left knee on towel and support body weight by placing hands on right thigh. Keep back straight. Slide hip towards until stretch is felt. Repeat ten times with each leg.

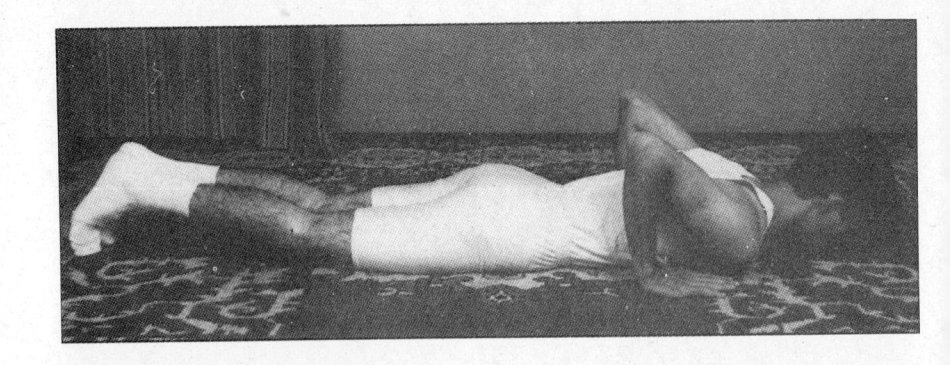

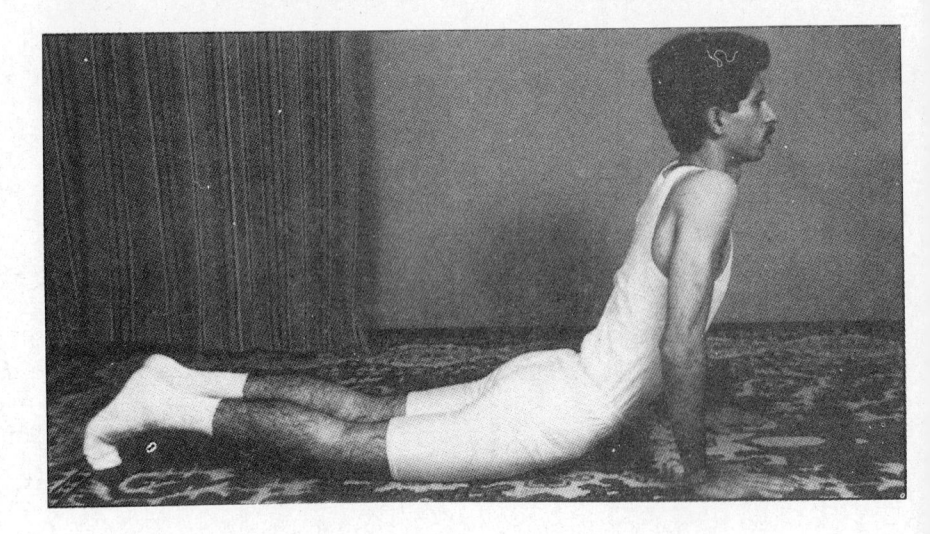

Press-ups:

Lie on stomach. Use arms to slowly raise the shoulders. Then straighten arms completely to produce advanced extension at the lumbar region. Count ten and then slowly relax. To start with, this exercise should be done only five times. (In vernacular language this exercise is also known as Bhujangasan or Sarpasan).

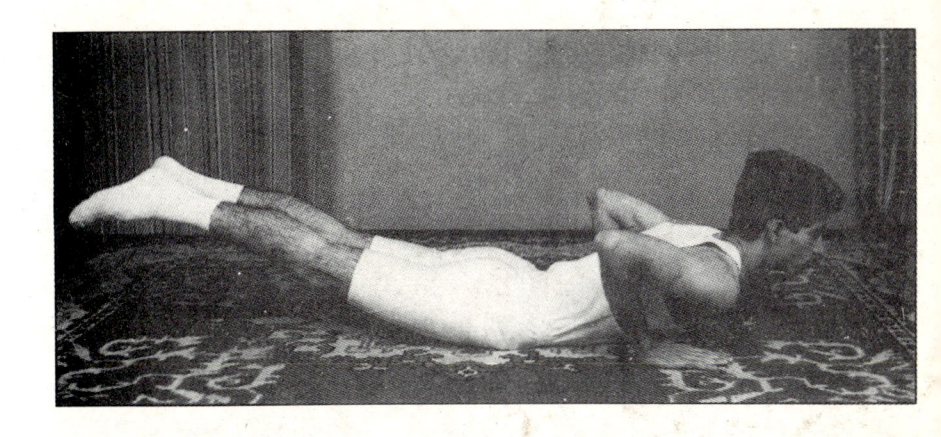

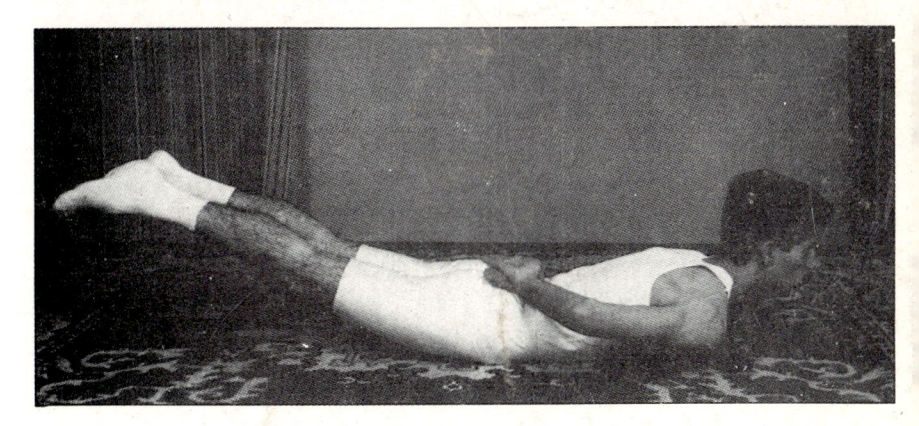

Shalabhasan or Intermediate Spinal Extension:

Lie on stomach. Use arms to slowly raise shoulders and then slowly raise the legs stretched without bending at the knees. Count ten. Do this exercise ten times.

Then repeat the above exercise by keeping the arms over the back and then simultaneously raising the head and lifting both legs by contracting the buttocks.

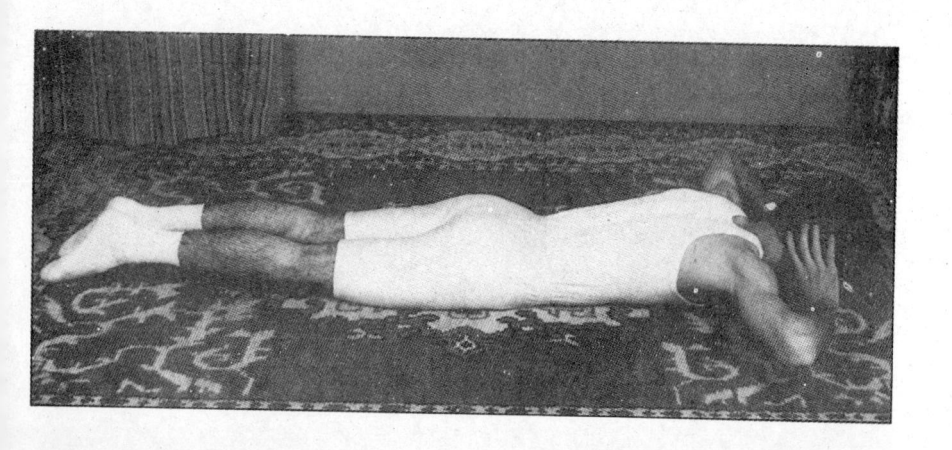

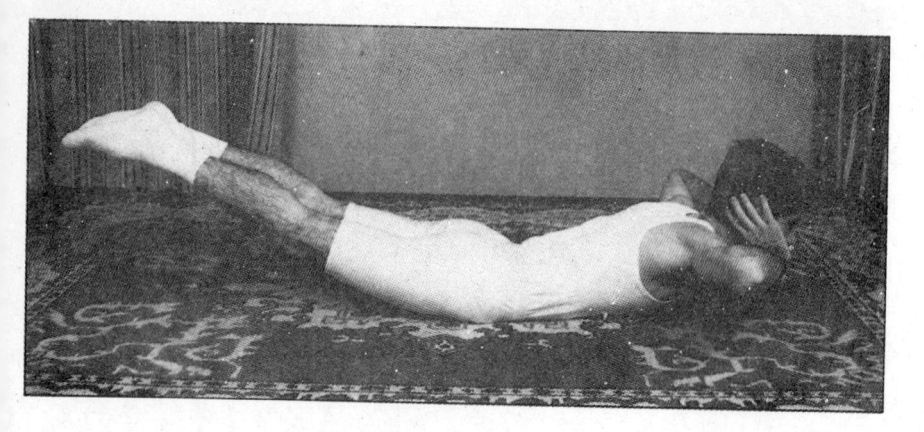

Advanced Spinal Extension:

Lie face down on stomach with elbows bent and fingers lightly touching the ears. Raise head and the upper body and breathe out at the same time.

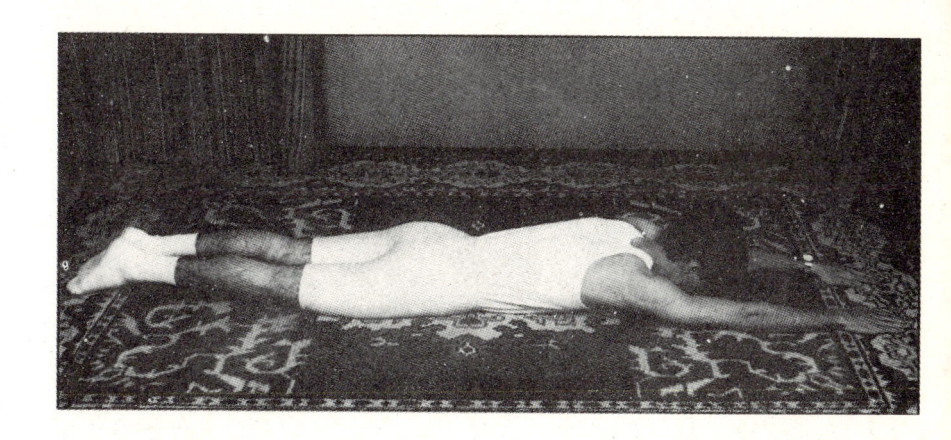

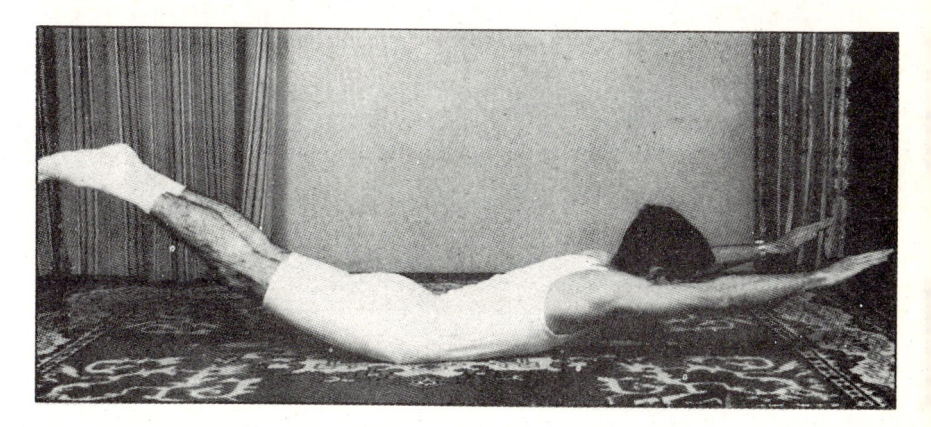

Advanced Spinal Extension:

Then once again lie face down relaxed. Stretch both arms above the head. Then raise head and upper body while breathing out and at the same time raise both legs by contracting the buttocks. This is in fact more advanced version of Shalabhasan.

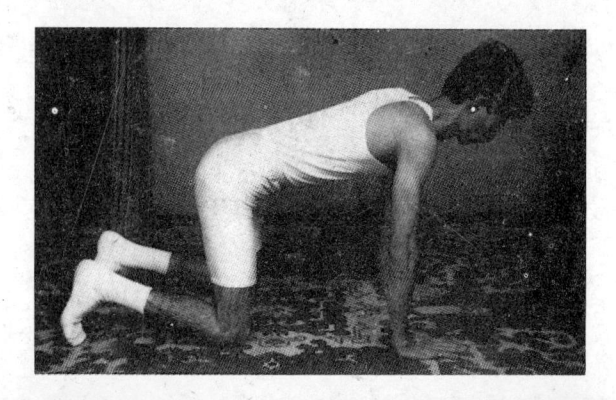

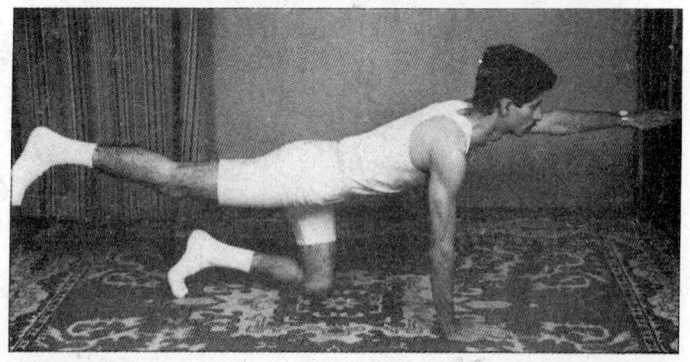

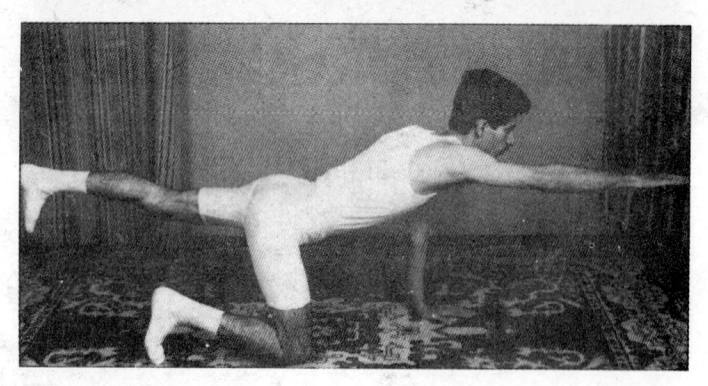

Quadriceps Exercises:

Lie on the floor like horse supporting the body on knees and arms. Then extend right arm at the level of head. Extend left leg and count ten. Repeat the exercise by stretching left arm and right leg. Repeat ten times.

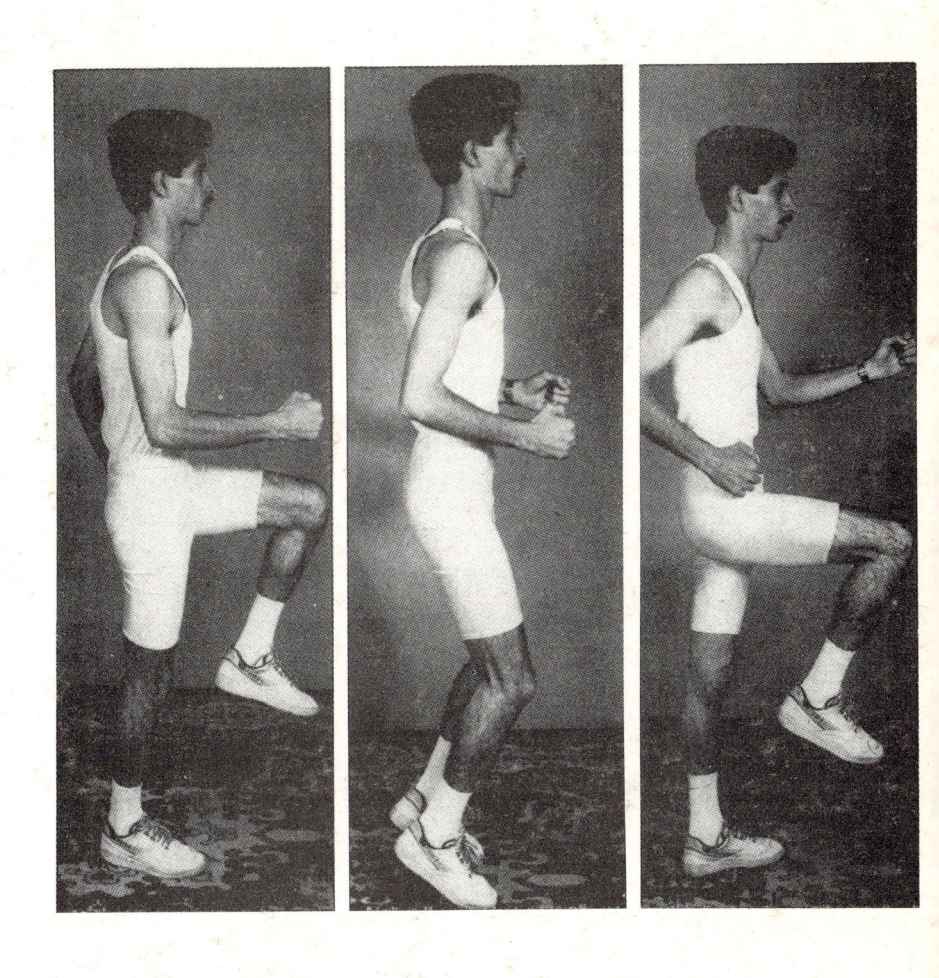

Jogging either in the garden or in the house is a good cardio-pulmonary exercise to increase the heart rate.

Cardio-pulmonary Exercise:

It is important to increase the efficiency of the heart and the lungs so that they can deliver the much needed energy and oxygen to the muscles which are doing exercise. A light jog or brisk walk can accomplish this. Walking is particularly easy for those just recovering from back sprains. Emphasis here is on duration and not intensity. A brisk walk for 20 minutes or a slow jog for a longer period of time is preferable to a short quick run. The ultimate goal is to raise the heart rate to a plateau at least three times in a week. Without going into too many details the plateau pulse for middle aged persons could be between 130 to 150 and for younger people it could be between 163 to 185 per minute. This activity tones up the heart and builds better power in the lungs to transport oxygen up to the blood.

How to Check the Heart Rate:

This is rather a difficult subject. Immediately after completing the exercise the pulse should be counted for ten seconds and then multiplied by six. Pulse can be easily felt at the carotid artery in the neck but this should not be the mode as pressure on the carotid artery may cause slowing of the heart rate.

Measuring the heart rate at the wrist on the radial artery may not be always successful as the artery may not be easily and quickly felt. It requires practice.

If measuring the pulse is difficult then one cay try "Walk test". If after a period of brisk walk one cannot say five words without taking a deep breath then the intensity of the exercise is great and should be decreased.

Once the exercise intensity reaches 80 per cent of one's capacity then endorphins are secreted in the blood giving the beneficial effect of masking the pain and showing euphoria.

The Cool Down:

After cardio-pulmonary exercise one should allow oneself to cool down. This prevents blood from pooling into the legs and causing dizziness. The cool down should last for a minimum period of three minutes. A longer cool down is needed for a more vigorous exercise. The cool down is complete when the heart rate has returned to below 100 beats a minute. Therapeutic exercises are now established as an important aspect of treatment of backpain and sciatica.

How to Take Care of Your
BACK

By following the instructions in this book, it is hoped, one will have achieved healthy spine away from aches and pains that one usually complains after the middle age and will pass through a phase in life of many years of pain free strong spine in good shape.

Other Important Books from UBSPD

GETTING PREGNANT
A Guide for the Infertile Couple

Dr. Aniruddha Malpani, et al

This comprehensive, but easy-to-understand, book offers new hope for those couples who are victims of infertility. The authors explain clearly and lucidly what infertility is; how it is caused; how it can be treated; and how infertile couples can cope with it effectively.

The book focuses on the latest techniques for determining the cause of, and effectively dealing with, infertility. The most important point that this book seeks to drive home is that the infertile patients (male or female) *should not* lose hope and *should actively* participate in their medical treatment.

AYURVEDA FOR HEALTHY LIVING

Dr. T L Devaraj

In this book, an attempt is made to emphasise *Shodhana* therapy which is one of the most important and advanced techniques of Ayurveda. It is unique as it can be used for preventing the disease, curing it and at the same time rejuvenating the body by increasing the immunity against the disease-producing organisms.

How to Maintain
GOOD HEALTH

Dr. B. M. Hegde

This Book provides a veritable treasure trove of information about various disorders and their prevention, control or cure along with the role of modern drugs. Also provides insights into the overall effects of factors such as food consumption patterns, exercise, smoking and alcohol intake on an individual's health. The book would prove to be a compact and useful source for *maintaining good health* for both the young and the old alike.

COMMON SEXUAL PROBLEMS
and Solutions

Dr. Prakash Kothari

"The book covers every man's and every woman's most important questions and concerns regarding their sex life...

-- Prof. John Money
The John Hopkins University, USA

With the help of this book, the reader can solve his problem without consulting a doctor...

-- *United News of India (UNI)*

all you need to know about
HAIR, SKIN & BEAUTY CARE

Blossom Kochhar

This is A COMPLETE BODY BOOK for all women who today, more than ever before, are aware of the need for looking good. It is compact, easy-to-understand and very practical. Three broad segments constitute the contents of the book. First, dedicated to grooming and upkeep of hair, second, exclusively to skin care and third, to the care of your body. The Body Care Section is dedicated to the hand and feet care and the figure upkeep for women.

Health & Beauty Through
AROMATHERAPY

Blossom Kochhar

The book is a complete guide to aromatherapy. It lists various oils, their uses and their medical application for ailments ranging from diabetes and arthritis to insomnia and depression. It also offers a beauty regimen and tips for dealing with problems such as cellulitis, pimples, ageing skin and falling hair.

STRETCH
yourself for
HEALTH & FITNESS

Bob Anderson

STRETCHING is the fastest growing type of exercise today. It helps keep your mind and body fit and simply makes you feel good. With over 1000 drawings and clear concise instructions, this book, considered a bible of the stretching gospel, of which over one million copies have already sold worldwide, will teach you the right way to stretch and help you to begin a regular, life-long programme of physical fitness.

A valuable contribution to the health and fitness field, experts recommend that "everyone should own and use this book".

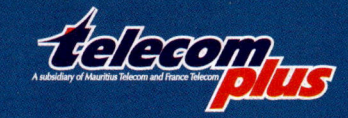

telecom plus
A subsidiary of Mauritius Telecom and France Telecom

Voici tout ce que NetPlus vous offre :

- Un **ordinateur haut de gamme**

Hewlett Packard multimédia avec

- **3 ans de garantie** et **livraison à domicile**

- **Abonnement Internet gratuit** jusqu'à fin décembre 2000

- **Formation Internet** à l'Espace Multimédia de Port Louis

- **1 adresse e-mail** (capacité 6Mo)

- 20Mo d'espace pour votre **page personnelle**

Caractéristiques techniques de l'ordinateur:
• Intel Pentium 466 MHz • 64 Mo SDRAM • 4.3 G.B disque dur • Système multimédia avec haut-parleurs • Modem interne de 56 K • Ecran couleur 15" SVGA • Windows 98

offre valable jusquà fin février 2000

Pour plus de renseignement, contactez Telecom Plus Ltd. , rez-de-chaussée, Telecom Tower, rue Edith Cavell, Port Louis. Tel . 203 7272 E-mail: servihoo@intnet.mu

L'accès Internet Complet

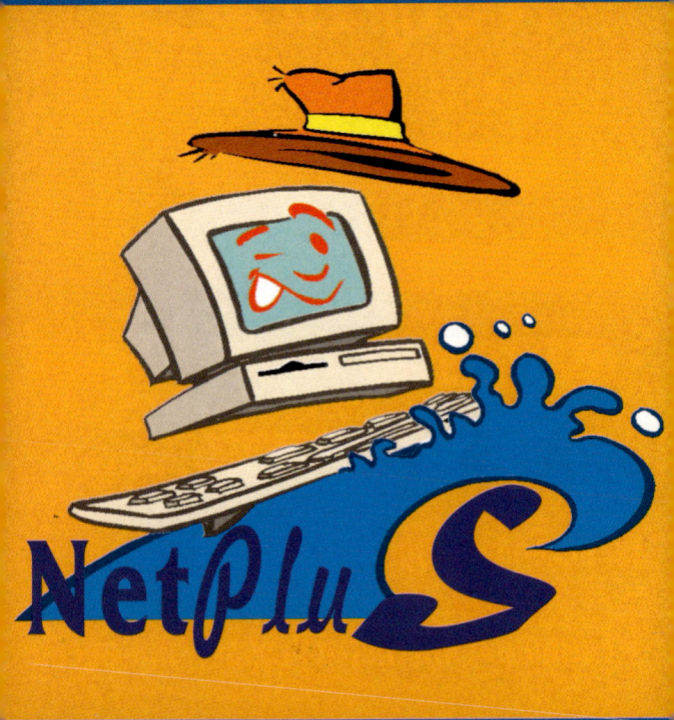

NetPlus

le super-pack PC plus Internet à un prix plus qu'abordable !

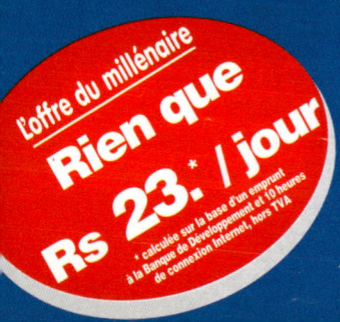

L'offre du millénaire
Rien que Rs 23.* / jour

* calculée sur la base d'un emprunt à la Banque de Développement et 10 heures de connexion Internet, hors TVA

telecom plus
A subsidiary of Mauritius Telecom and France Telecom

YOGA
FOR CHILDREN
A Complete Illustrated Guide to Yoga
including a Manual for Parents and Teachers

Swati Chanchani
Rajiv Chanchani

As yoga becomes more popular throughout the world, there is a pressing need for a good book on Yoga for children which is both authoritative and appealing, informative and enjoyable. The authors of this book fulfil this need admirably. They trace the roots of Yoga in mythology and legend, and include many stories and tales bringing out the quality of, and inspiration for, the postures. They also stress the links of the postures to the natural world -- trees, mountains, flowers, animals. They emphasise the universal moral and ethical values implicit in the practice of Yoga such as non-violence, truth, self-discipline, simplicity, and contentment. Besides they highlight the geometrical forms and precision in the postures, so that children can relate to these abstract concepts through what they have learnt in their body movements.

Each Yoga postures is explained through photographs, drawings, stories and detailed instructions with stick figures illustrating several stages in performing the pose. Important "dos and don'ts" and the benefits of each pose are also given.

The highlight of the book is a detailed section meant for parents and teachers comprising specific guidance on keeping children practising Yoga creatively, enjoyably and safely.

Three Bestsellers from UBSPD

how to control your
BLOOD PRESSURE
for healthy living
Dr. G. D. Thapar

This extremely useful book has been written, for the layperson, in a simple and lucid style, keeping medical terminology and theories to the minimum.

LIFE AFTER 50
Dr. G. D. Thapar

Based on simple, commonsense principles of health, the book presents in an easy-to-understand language the body changes that occur with age and explains, how, in the light of those changes, adjustments in diet, work, exercise, rest, etc., have to be made. It also goes on to explain disorders common at this age -- obesity, stress, diabetes, high blood pressure, heart attacks, strokes, cancer, enlarged prostate, Parkinson's disease, etc and how to prevent and steer clear of them.

all you need to know about
HEART ATTACKS
Dr. G. D. Thapar

This simply and concisely written book, aimed at the general public, contains useful information pertaining to heart attacks...The author must be praised for his simple, No-nonsense style of handling instructions pertaining to first-aid in a cardiac arrest. Supported by good illustrations, the step-by-step instructions on mouth to mouth breathing and external cardiac massage make excellent reading.

Also Available!

all you need to know about the
CARE OF YOUR TEETH
(Your Complete Tooth and Gum Care Guide)

Dr. Arun Kumar

This Book has been prepared to help you understand some of the problems that occur in your mouth; how modern dentistry can help you; what preventive measures you should take. It answers the most common questions that you may ask. This book is also meant to demystify a great deal of apprehension and allay common fears associated with dentistry. A **MUST** for all of you.

---

all you need to know about
BABY AND CHILD CARE

Dr. Rajesh N. Kumar

This Book is written to help you care for your child -- the advice is from the time he or she is born right through adolescence. All the subjects and problems that cause frequent concerns have been covered in detail.

This exceptionally easy-to-refer guide is a MUST for every parent, guardian and caretaker.

Other Important Books from UBSPD

Anderson, B	Stretch Yourself for Health and Fitness
Chanchani, R	Yoga for Children
Devaraj, T L Dr	Ayurveda for Healthy Living
Kochhar, B	Health and Beauty Through Aromatherapy
Kochhar, B	All You Need to Know About Hair, Skin and Beauty Care
Kothari, P Dr.	Common Sexual Problems and their Solutions
Kumar, A Dr.	All You Need to Know About the Care of Your Teeth
Kumar, R	All You Need to Know About Baby and Child Care
Malpani	Getting Pregnant: A Guide for the Infertile Couple
Ramani, P S	All You Need to Know About Pain in Your Neck
Singh, Rahul	Family Planning Success Stories
Thapar, G D Dr.	All You Need to Know About Heart Attacks
Thapar, G D Dr.	How to Control Your Blood Pressure
Thapar, G D Dr.	Life After 50
Thapar, G D Dr.	Stay Healthy with Diabetes
Ahuja, M R	Cancer : Causes & Prevention
Gupta, A Dr.	How to Control Asthma